WITHDRAWN
WRIGHT STATE UNIVERSITY LIBRARIES

DATE DUE

MAY

The Diagnosis and Treatment of Drug and Alcohol Abuse

Sidney Cohen, MD, DSc, has written 285 articles, chapters and books on substance abuse. He is a Clinical Professor of Psychiatry at the Neuropsychiatric Institute, UCLA School of Medicine and has served as Director of the Division of Narcotic Addiction and Drug Abuse, NIMH. He consults for many organizations including the State Department, the FDA, the Army and is on the National Advisory Council of the NIDA. He has received numerous honors and awards including the first Sidney Cohen Lectureship in Substance Abuse Medicine.

Dr. James Callahan holds a doctorate in Public Administration from the University of Southern California. He has served as Deputy Director of the Division of Training of the National Institute on Drug Abuse (NIDA), and as Director of NIDA's Medical and Health Professions Education Program. He has also served as a member of the White House Task Force on Prescribing, and the American Medical Association (AMA) Informal Steering Committee on Prescription Drug Abuse. He is currently Director of Smoking Research Application for the National Cancer Institute's Division of Cancer Prevention and Control.

The Diagnosis and Treatment of Drug and Alcohol Abuse

Editor
Sidney Cohen, MD

Consulting Editor
James F. Callahan, DPA

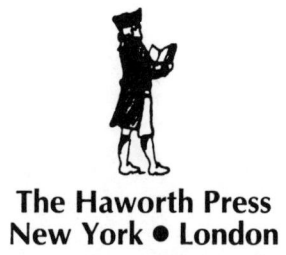

The Haworth Press
New York • London

RC
564
.D53
1986

© 1986 by The Haworth Press, Inc. All rights reserved. No part of this work may be reproduced or utilized in any form or by any means, electronic or mechanical, including photocopying, microfilm and recording, or by any information storage and retrieval system, without permission in writing from the publisher. Printed in the United States of America.

The Haworth Press, Inc., 28 East 22 Street, New York, New York 10010-6194
EUROSPAN/Haworth, 3 Henrietta Street, London WC2E 8LU England

Earlier versions of most of the chapters in this book were published in *Diagnosis of Drug and Alcohol Abuse* by S. Cohen and D. M. Gallant, Medical Monograph Series Vol. 1., No. 6, and *Treatment of Drug and Alcohol Abuse* by D. C. Lewis and E. C. Senay, Medical Monograph Series, Vol. II, No. 2, Career Teacher Center, State University of New York, Downstate Medical Center, Brooklyn, New York, 1981.

Library of Congress Cataloging in Publication Data
Main entry under title:

The Diagnosis and treatment of drug and alcohol abuse.

    Includes bibliographies and index.
    1. Drug abuse. 2. Alcoholism. I. Cohen, Sidney, 1910–   . II. Callahan, James F.
[DNLM: 1. Alcoholism—diagnosis. 2. Alcoholism—therapy. 3. Substance Abuse—diagnosis. 4. Substance Abuse—therapy.
WM 270 D536]
RC564.D53   1986   616.86'3   85-24833
ISBN 0-86656-479-9

Contents

Introduction		ix
Acknowledgments		xi
1	**Diagnosis Pretest**	**1**
	Diagnosis Pretest Answer Key 9	
2	**Introduction to Diagnosis**	**11**
	Use of Terms 12	
	Confidentiality 13	
3	**The Patient Interview**	**15**
	Orientation to the Patient 15	
	The Personal History Interview 18	
4	**The Physical Examination**	**33**
	Signs and Symptoms of Drug and Alcohol Abuse 33	
5	**Diagnosis of Medical Complications of Alcohol and Drug Abuse**	**39**
	Medical Complications of Drug and Alcohol Abuse 39	
	Complications Unrelated to Drug Abuse 57	
	Maternal and Neonatal Complications 58	
6	**Helpful Diagnostic Tests**	**63**
	Testing with Naloxone 63	
	Test for Alcohol Dependence 65	
	Laboratory Tests 66	
	Considerations for Evaluation 67	
7	**Diagnosis Posttest**	**69**
	Diagnosis Posttest Answer Key 77	

8	**Treatment Pretest**	79
	Treatment Pretest Answer Key *90*	

9	**Responding to Common Emergencies**	93
	General Management of Crisis *93*	
	Behavioral Emergencies *94*	
	Observation and Diagnosis *98*	
	Management of Shock *99*	
	Hyperventilation *100*	

10	**A General Approach to the Comatose and Semicomatose Patient**	103
	The Comatose Patient *103*	
	Management of Convulsions *107*	
	The Semicomatose Patient *109*	
	Management of Orally Ingested Drugs *109*	

11	**A Specific Approach to the Treatment of Drug and Alcohol Abusing Patients**	115
	Opiate Overdose *115*	
	Opiate Withdrawal *116*	
	Methadone Withdrawal *117*	
	Alcohol Overdose *118*	
	Alcohol Withdrawal *119*	
	Sedative-Hypnotic and Minor-Tranquilizer Overdose *121*	
	Sedative-Hypnotic and Minor-Tranquilizer Withdrawal *122*	
	Other Treatment Approaches *124*	
	Abuse of Volatiles *126*	
	Stimulant Abuse *127*	
	Stimulant Withdrawal *128*	
	Hallucinogens *129*	
	Phencyclidine (PCP) Reactions *131*	
	Cannabis *134*	
	Multiple Drug Abuse *135*	

12	**Drug and Alcohol Related Problems in the Physician's Office**	137

13 Management of Opiate Dependent Patients in the General Hospital — 143
Methadone Maintenance Patients on the General Medical Ward   *143*
"Street Addicts" on the General Medical Ward   *145*
Surgery on the Drug and Alcohol Abuser   *148*
Analgesia for Drug Dependent Patients   *150*
Management of the Infant Withdrawal Syndrome   *151*
Alcoholics in the General Hospital   *151*

14 Pharmacotherapy of Drug and Alcohol Abusing Patients — 153
General Comments on Chemotherapy, Narcotic Addiction, and Alcoholism   *153*
Methadone Maintenance   *153*
Other Opioid Substitutes   *159*
Narcotic Antagonists   *160*
Antabuse (Disulfiram)   *161*
Other Drugs   *162*

15 Sociotherapy of Drug and Alcohol Abusers — 165
Therapeutic Communities   *165*
Modified Therapeutic Communities   *168*
Other Sociotherapies   *169*
AA, Al-Anon, and Alateen   *170*
Coercive Treatment   *171*

16 Experimental Treatment Modalities — 175
Transcendental Meditation   *175*
Biofeedback and Relaxation Techniques   *176*
Acupuncture and Behavior Modification   *176*
Clonidine in Opiate Withdrawal   *176*

17 Treatment Posttest — 179
Treatment Posttest Answer Key   *188*

Appendix A   Assessment Interviewing Guide — 191
I. Readiness   *191*
II. Relationships   *195*

III. Rationality *200*
IV. Resources *203*
Behavioral Assessment Inventory *209*

Appendix B   Quick Reference Guide to Intoxication, Withdrawal, Overdose, and Emergency Management   213

Drug and Alcohol Overdose and the Comatose Patient *213*
Fever of Unknown Origin in the Drug or Alcohol Abuser *214*
Helpful Diagnostic Aids *214*

Appendix C   Resources for Training the Physician and Health Professional in Drugs, Alcohol, and Prescribing: An Annotated Compendium   231

Introduction *231*
Medical and Health Professions Education in Drugs and Alcohol *232*
Prescribing *235*
Conclusion *236*

PART I: Drug and Alcohol Education Resources   238

Section One: Curricula and General Reviews of Education Resources *238*
Section Two: Clinical Manuals *245*
Section Three: Films and Videocassettes *249*
Section Four: Examinations and Certification Procedures *254*
Section Five: Organizations *256*

PART II: Prescribing, Dispensing, and Administering Controlled Substances   268

Section One: General Texts and Resources *268*
Section Two: Diversion for Purposes of Abuse *274*
Section Three: The Impaired Professional *280*
Section Four: State-wide Programs *285*

Index   **293**

Introduction

A quarter of adult deaths are substance abuse related, the great majority from alcohol and tobacco abuse, with other abused products making a more modest contribution at this time. Therefore, those who practice medicine and all its specialties are repeatedly concerned with the diagnosis and treatment of the diverse group of abused drugs that can induce a broad array of symptoms, signs, complications, and problems in management.

This book is written for every health professional who comes into contact with patients who have used legal or illegal agents unwisely. These contacts seem to be occurring more frequently at present. The book will serve as a text for some and as a reference work for others. We hope it meets your needs.

Particular attention is directed to Appendix C: Resources for Training the Physician and Health Professional in Drugs, Alcohol, and Prescribing: An Annotated Compendium. It is a resource that consolidates many different sources valuable in self-instruction or in teaching. Education resources, films and videocassettes, examinations and certification procedures, and selected clinical and research references appear in the compendium. Prescribing practice resources also are included. References to texts and organizations interested in the problem, prescribing for specific indication: pain, the elderly, alcohol as it relates to prescribing, and diversions of psychoactive drugs as they relate to physicians, pharmacists, and hospital personnel all are mentioned. References for the impaired physician, pharmacist, nurse, and dentist are included. State-wide education and enforcement programs and an AMA manual on establishing educational programs on prescribing and diversion complete the annotated compendium. It can be used to find out who to call for further information, what training aids and references are available, and to meet other needs that may arise.

Sidney Cohen, MD
James F. Callahan, DPA

Acknowledgments

This volume has brought up-to-date a number of monographs from the Medical Monograph Series issued by the National Institute on Drug Abuse. We express our appreciation to the National Institute on Drug Abuse and the following authors of the earlier editions.

Charles E. Becker, MD
Donald M. Gallant, MD
David C. Lewis, MD
Charles P. O'Brien, MD, PHD
Anthony E. Raynes, MD
Sidney H. Schnoll, MD
Edward C. Senay, MD
Donald R. Wesson, MD

1
Diagnosis Pretest

Answers to the Pretest appear on page 9.

PART I. TRUE-FALSE QUESTIONS
DIRECTIONS: For each statement below, place a check mark next to the "T" if the statement is true, or next to the "F" if it is false.

1. Repeated snorting of cocaine can result in a perforated cartilaginous nasal septum.

   T _____ F _____

2. Clinical signs of the neonate withdrawal syndrome almost always appear no later than a few days after birth.

   T _____ F _____

3. Continuous amphetamine use often heightens the drug's anorexigenic effects.

   T _____ F _____

4. Drug abuse can alter the requirements of hypertensive patients for their medication.

   T _____ F _____

5. An underlying psychotic condition should be considered when patients do not respond to drug abuse treatment interventions.

   T _____ F _____

6. The sedative effects of anticonvulsant medication used to control epilepsy may be diminished by abuse of certain drugs.

   T _____ F _____

7. Thrombophlebitis (when present) often occurs at the site of injection.

   T _____ F _____

8. Serum hepatitis is acquired only by the entry of the virus through broken skin.

   T _____ F _____

9. The naloxone test can be used to exclude the presence of physical dependence on opiates/opioids.

   T _____ F _____

10. The examining physician should avoid asking a patient directly about suicidal potential, as this is likely to plant the idea of suicide in his or her head.

    T _____ F _____

11. Aphasia is a disorder due to poor comprehension, symbolization, and reproduction of concepts during speech or writing.

    T _____ F _____

12. Chronic use of amphetamines is often characterized by stereotyped behavior, e.g., repeatedly picking at the skin.

    T _____ F _____

13. Impulse control is a good prognostic indicator for having the ability to complete treatment successfully.

    T _____ F _____

14. All patients entering a drug treatment program should be evaluated for venereal disease.

    T _____ F _____

15. The lifestyle of patients is of little importance to the development of the treatment plan.

    T _____   F _____

PART II. MULTIPLE CHOICE QUESTIONS
DIRECTIONS: Each question below has four or five answers. Pick the **one** answer to each question that is **most true** and place a check mark in front of that answer.

16. How long after last use do symptoms of withdrawal from morphine and heroin begin?

    _____ A. 2-4 hours.
    _____ B. 6-12 hours.
    _____ C. 12-14 hours.
    _____ D. 24-48 hours.
    _____ E. 48-60 hours.

17. Which of the following is true about the use of depressants?

    _____ A. Inability to attain orgasm may result, but **only** if use is chronic and in high doses.
    _____ B. Even small doses may produce impotence in males.
    _____ C. Use does not affect orgasmic functions in women.
    _____ D. All of the above are true.
    _____ E. None of the above is true.

18. Severe pain is likely to result from—
    _____ A. Cutaneous injection of heroin.
    _____ B. Oral ingestion of stimulants.
    _____ C. Subcutaneous injection of stimulants.
    _____ D. Intraarterial injection.

19. The withdrawal syndrome of neonates born to mothers addicted to opiates/opioids—

    _____ A. Is the least significant neonatal complication.
    _____ B. Applies only to the babies of mothers addicted to heroin.

4 / *The Diagnosis and Treatment of Drug and Alcohol Abuse*

    ____ C. Happens only when the mother is undergoing withdrawal within a few days of giving birth.

    ____ D. None of the above is true.

20. A detailed sexual history assessing development and current status—

    ____ A. Is desirable but not very important.

    ____ B. Should usually be obtained late in treatment.

    ____ C. Should usually be obtained some time early in treatment.

    ____ D. Should always be obtained by some staff member other than a physician.

21. Which cardiovascular complication is most serious and prevalent among heroin users?

    ____ A. Hypertension.

    ____ B. Myocardial disease.

    ____ C. Infective endocarditis.

    ____ D. Cardiac arrhythmias.

    ____ E. All are equally prevalent.

Pick the **one** answer to each question below that is **not** true and place a check mark in front of the answer.

22. Which **one** of the following is **not** true?

    ____ A. Withdrawal from meprobamate can produce convulsions within the first few days.

    ____ B. Withdrawal from diazepam produces convulsions on the first day.

    ____ C. At least 75 mg of chlordizepoxide daily for 2 months is required to produce dependency.

    ____ D. Physical dependence on pentobarbital has been demonstrated.

23. Which of the following is **not** a frequent sign of infective endocarditis in a drug abuser?

    ____ A. High white cell count.

    ____ B. Fever of unknown origin.

Diagnosis Pretest / 5

_____ C. Pneumonia.
_____ D. Embolic phenomena.

24. Which **one** of the following is **not** associated with long-term drug abuse?

    _____ A. Infections in the lung.
    _____ B. Tuberculosis.
    _____ C. Spontaneous pneumothorax.
    _____ D. Foreign body granulomas in the lungs.

PART III. MATCHING QUESTIONS

A. DIRECTIONS: For each numbered set of symptoms, signs, and diagnostic indicators given below, select the **one** lettered heading that **most** closely applies and place a check mark in front of the corresponding letter.

    A. Withdrawal from stimulants
    B. Intoxication with depressants
    C. Intoxication with PCP
    D. Intoxication with opiates/opioids
    E. Intoxication with stimulants

25. Sleepiness, feeling of floating, pinpoint pupils.

    _____ A _____ B _____ C _____ D _____ E

26. Apathy, hyperphagia, hypersomnia.

    _____ A _____ B _____ C _____ D _____ E

27. Anxiety, euphoria, anorexia.

    _____ A _____ B _____ C _____ D _____ E

28. Blank stare, hypertension, nystagmus.

    _____ A _____ B _____ C _____ D _____ E

29. Hypertension, elevated heart rate, stereotyped behavior

    _____ A _____ B _____ C _____ D _____ E

30. Delirium, elevated heart rate, tremor.

   ____ A   ____ B   ____ C   ____ D   ____ E

31. Hypotonia, ataxia, nystagmus.

   ____ A   ____ B   ____ C   ____ D   ____ E

32. Irritability, sluggishness, poor judgment.

   ____ A   ____ B   ____ C   ____ D   ____ E

33. General fatigue, hypersomnia, apathy.

   ____ A   ____ B   ____ C   ____ D   ____ E

34. Slurred speech, dysarthria, floating feeling.

   ____ A   ____ B   ____ C   ____ D   ____ E

35. Hypertension, facial grimacing, vomiting.

   ____ A   ____ B   ____ C   ____ D   ____ E

36. Anorexia, tactile hallucinations, irritability.

   ____ A   ____ B   ____ C   ____ D   ____ E

B. DIRECTIONS: For each numbered set of symptoms, signs, and diagnostic indicators given below select the **one** lettered heading that **most** closely applies and place a check mark in front of the corresponding letter.

   A. Overdose of stimulants
   B. Intoxication with hallucinogens
   C. Withdrawal from opiates/opioids
   D. Withdrawal from depressants

37. Tactile hallucinations, hypertension, insomnia.

   ____ A   ____ B   ____ C   ____ D

38. Visual hallucinations, anorexia, synesthesia, labile affect.

   ____ A   ____ B   ____ C   ____ D

39. Orthostatic hypotension, psychosis.

　　____ A 　　____ B 　　____ C 　　____ D

40. Irritability, anorexia, coryza.

　　____ A 　　____ B 　　____ C 　　____ D

41. Chest pain, anxiety, diarrhea.

　　____ A 　　____ B 　　____ C 　　____ D

PART IV. MULTIPLE TRUE AND FALSE
DIRECTIONS: Each of the following items has four choices, one of which may be correct, two of which may be correct, three of which may be correct, or all of which may be correct. Using the following key, place the appropriate letter in front of each of the following numbered items.

　　A.　Only 1, 2, and 3 are correct
　　B.　Only 1 and 3 are correct
　　C.　Only 2 and 4 are correct
　　D.　Only 4 is correct
　　E.　All are correct

		DIRECTIONS SUMMARIZED		
A	B	C	D	E
1,2,3 only	1,3 only	2,4 only	4 only	All are correct

____ 42. Which of the following septic problem(s) is (are) associated with drug abuse?

　　(1) Foul-smelling discharge.
　　(2) Gas formation.
　　(3) Stony or wooden-hard tenseness.
　　(4) Cellulitis or fasciolitis.

____ 43. Which of the following can be associated with alcohol abuse?

(1) Tachycardia.
(2) Acne rosacea.
(3) Spider nevi.
(4) Bullae.

____ 44. The inability to achieve orgasm may result from chronic high dosages of—

(1) Stimulants.
(2) Depressants.
(3) PCP.
(4) Alcohol.

____ 45. Nystagmus can occur during—

(1) Alcohol withdrawal.
(2) PCP intoxication.
(3) Depressant intoxication.
(4) Stimulant withdrawal.

____ 46. Neonate withdrawal syndrome is most associated with—

(1) Stimulants.
(2) Depressants.
(3) PCP.
(4) Opiates.

____ 47. Which of the following signs is associated with **low-dose** phencyclidine (PCP) intoxication?

(1) Drooling.
(2) Tachycardia.
(3) Muscle rigidity.
(4) Increased deep tendon reflexes.

____ 48. In the nonintravenous user, which of the following is associated with fever of unknown origin (FUO)?

(1) Alcohol and drug withdrawal states (e.g., delirium tremens).

(2) Hepatitis.
(3) Acute drug reactions.
(4) Tuberculosis.

___ 49. For which of the following may the EEG be a useful diagnostic aid?

(1) Stimulant withdrawal.
(2) Hallucinogen withdrawal.
(3) Sedative-hypnotic withdrawal.
(4) Opiate withdrawal.

___ 50. Which of the following tests should be performed when evaluating a patient for possible treatment in a drug abuse program?

(1) SMA-12.
(2) CBC.
(3) Urine screen.
(4) Australia antigen.

DIAGNOSIS PRETEST ANSWER KEY

Answer	Answer
1. T	26. A
2. F	27. E
3. F	28. C
4. T	29. E
5. T	30. E
6. F	31. B
7. T	32. B
8. F	33. A

DIAGNOSIS PRETEST ANSWER KEY (continued)

Answer	Answer
9. T	34. B
10. F	35. C
11. T	36. E
12. T	37. A
13. T	38. B
14. T	39. D
15. F	40. C
16. B	41. A
17. A	42. E
18. D	43. A
19. D	44. E
20. C	45. A
21. C	46. C
22. B	47. C
23. A	48. A
24. C	49. B
25. D	50. E

2
Introduction to Diagnosis

This chapter is designed to provide the health professional with a concise and thorough discussion of the drug and/or alcohol abusing patient. The assessment of this patient is complicated by many problems which are peculiar to a substance abuse population—specific problems not usually encountered with other patients. The psychological, social, and medical manifestations of substance abuse vary widely, depending on the particular substance of abuse, the degree of involvement with it, and a wide variety of other circumstances in the patient's life. This volume focuses on these specific problems and on diagnostic methods which will aid the health professional in assessing the patient. The ultimate goal of this process of diagnosing the drug or alcohol abusing patient is the development of an effective treatment plan for that individual.

To encompass the wide range of information, the basic approach to diagnosis has been divided into four major sections: The Patient Interview, The Physical Examination, Diagnosis of Medical Complications of Drug and Alcohol Abuse, and Helpful Diagnostic Tests.

The patient interview. Interviewing the drug or alcohol abusing patient does, by necessity, differ from conducting a traditional interview. Inquiry into the patient's lifestyle must include considering his or her drug and/or alcohol history, social adjustment, sexual functioning, psychological status, education, and employment history, as well as any criminal background and/or record of arrest.

The physical examination. The physical examination must not only yield the usual information about the patient, but must also yield information about such special factors as the many signs and symptoms of alcohol and drug abuse, associated medical complications, and existing medical conditions that can be complicated by substance abuse.

Diagnosis of medical complications of drug and alcohol abuse. The medical complications arising from drug and alcohol abuse pose a serious challenge to the physician who must understand not only the physical effects of drugs, but also the circumstances in which specific drugs are taken. Complications may range from mild to serious and affect various organ systems. Subtle signs and symptoms may often go unnoticed by both the patient and the unaware physician. A vast array of physical abnormalities are either caused by or exacerbated by drug use. Specific diagnostic techniques are presented which can be used to assess physical status. With effective interviewing and examination many, if not all, medical complications can be recognized and treated.

Helpful diagnostic tests. Because of the medical complications commonly observed in substance abusing patients, a complete battery of diagnostic tests is indicated whenever drug or alcohol abuse is suspected. These tests should consist of a urine analysis (including a drug screen), blood studies such as the SMA-12 and SMA-6, and, in some cases, an EKG, EEG, Pap smear, pregnancy test, and blood alcohol level.

Although the emphasis of the material in this monograph is on full-scale diagnosis and evaluation, a Quick Reference Guide appears in this monograph in Appendix B, which outlines signs, symptoms, and diagnostic aids for intoxication, withdrawal, and overdose. The first page of the Quick Reference Guide includes standard procedures for managing the emergency patient.

USE OF TERMS

For the purpose of clarity and to avoid misunderstanding or misinterpretation of terminology, the following definitions are supplied.

Detoxification refers to the treatment of physical dependence by giving gradually reduced doses of the drug on which the person is dependent or of a drug that has cross-tolerance with the original drug. Detoxification is not considered to be a definitive treatment, because almost all patients who are simply detoxified without follow-up including psychosocial rehabilitation will relapse very soon after having been discharged. Thus, detoxification should be regarded only as the initial phase in a definitive treatment program.

Drug dependence has been used instead of "addiction," and wherever possible the type of drug dependence has been specified; e.g., alcohol dependence, heroin dependence, or amphetamine dependence.

Wherever the word "dependence" is used, it refers either to physical dependence, psychological dependence, or both.

Methadone is a long-acting synthetic narcotic that may be taken orally and is used in detoxification from opiate dependence as well as in methadone maintenance. Wherever the detrimental effects of methadone are mentioned in this text, it should be understood that the reference applies to methadone obtained illicitly and/or administered without supervision, not to methadone that is administered under medical supervision for the purposes of either detoxification or maintenance.

Rehabilitation refers to the process of providing vocational, educational, and social services in conjunction with medical and/or psychological treatment.

The distinction between *short-term* and *long-term treatment* lies primarily in the goals of treatment. In this context, short-term treatment refers to the initial steps which provide a basis for the later long-term goals. For example, if long-term goals for the patient are to be alcohol- and/or drug-free, make educational progress, and obtain employment, then short-term treatment might include the provision of detoxification, counseling to explore vocational interests, and skill-training opportunities. Although in some cases the terms might be used to differentiate the duration and extent of treatment (e.g., detoxification versus social rehabilitation), it is assumed that most readers will be addressing a broad range of patients' needs that encompass both short-term and long-term goals.

Signs are the *objective* indicators of a disease and are perceptible to the examining person; e.g., rash, rapid pulse, etc. *Symptoms* are the *subjective* sensations a patient reports to the examining physician; e.g., nausea, headache, anxiety, etc.

CONFIDENTIALITY

Stringent laws control the use and disclosure of information gathered and recorded about alcohol and drug abusing patients in treatment programs. All treatment program personnel—physicians, nurses, counselors, secretaries, etc.—should be familiar with these regulations. Physicians especially must be alert to the restrictions concerning the disclosure of patient information. We urge physicians to study these regulations to determine their liability under both federal and state confidentiality rules and regulations. One aid available for studying the confidentiality regulations is the course "Confidentiality of Alcohol and Drug Abuse Patient Records," which may be ordered from the National Clearinghouse for Drug Abuse Information, P.O.B. 416, Kensington, MD 20795.

3
The Patient Interview

ORIENTATION TO THE PATIENT

Physicians frequently fail to recognize and diagnose drug and alcohol abusers. Jones's (1979) study of a psychiatric emergency clinic reported that one-half of the alcoholic patients seen in that clinic were not diagnosed by the admitting physician. In addition to focusing on the diagnosis of drug and alcohol abuse, this section is intended to help the physician assess and understand the unique set of problems, circumstances, and resources the patient brings to the treatment situation.

In order for the physician to achieve an understanding of the patient's lifestyle and resources, techniques must be used that will elicit information from the patient in a focused, well-organized interview. Before reviewing the specific elements of the interview strategy, some widely held assumptions about drug and alcohol abusing patients should be mentioned.

1. Although the patient is often categorized as having a "junkie" or "user" personality, there is no consistent personality type that fits all substance abusers. Each patient is unique, at least from the viewpoint of his or her experiences, both before and after becoming drug or alcohol dependent.
2. Consideration of the psychology and sociology of the individual patient requires a careful distinction being made between cause and effect. For example, it is known that certain drugs promote passivity and psychological dependence. It does not logically follow, however, that every drug abuser is a passive-dependent individual, or that passive-dependent types are good candidates for drug abuse.
3. Drug and alcohol users and abusers have various reasons for their behavior; e.g., psychiatric problems, external problems, or

pleasure seeking. An analysis of these reasons helps determine the patient's strengths and weaknesses, thus serving as an indicator of the potential success or failure in a given treatment schedule.
4. If environmental or external pressures are identified as the primary causes of abuse (note the instance of some drug dependent military personnel in Vietnam), removal of these pressures or learning how to deal with stress is one approach to treatment. Treatment experience indicates that such an approach is possible, but caution is required. Other treatment efforts may also be necessary.
5. There is no single type of program that is right for all substance dependent individuals. Psychiatric or internal problems (e.g., self-destructive or acting-out behavior, inconsistency in thought and behavior, strong dependency needs, or inability to defer gratification or delay impulses) cause some patients to fail to respond to treatment in a program that may have proved successful for others. Such failures tend to reinforce whatever feelings of low self-esteem the patient may already possess. Each patient is unique and therefore requires an individualized, personally tailored treatment plan.

The therapeutic techniques necessary to treat the substance abuser require much more than being supportive, acting as an advocate, or treating the patient as simply being a medical problem. The initial interview may be the most critical encounter for ensuring that the drug or alcohol abusing patient will receive the future treatment necessary to live a drug-free existence. The success of this interview depends to a great extent on the physician's skill in creating an atmosphere of trust, his or her awareness of the possibility of covert or unintentional abuse, and the ability to confront this issue in a forthright but nonjudgmental manner. Some substance abusers present themselves for treatment of their drug or alcohol problem, but far more commonly conceal such problems from the physician or deny it to themselves. In such cases, the method chosen to confront this possibility may be crucial to ensuring further treatment. The physician must be particularly sensitive to this patient and convey the feeling that he or she cares about the individual.

No matter how much a patient denies drug or alcohol use and abuse during the course of a clinical interview, certain signs, symptoms, and behaviors will indicate the opposite to the alert physician. The following are some of the more common indicators:

1. Physical findings seriously out of proportion to the patient's complaints.
2. A history of trauma, including burns and broken bones that occur with a higher frequency than would normally be expected given the occupation and activities of the patient.
3. Single-auto accidents, especially more than two such accidents in a short time period.
4. Seizures, especially when they appear for the first time between the ages of 10 and 30.
5. Drastic shifts in a patient's level of functioning.
6. Excessive interest in drugs on the part of a patient.
7. Demands by the patient for specific drugs or increased drug dosages.

The diagnosis of a drug or alcohol abuse problem is especially critical when certain classes of drugs may be indicated for the treatment of a patient (for example, anticoagulants).

In some instances, the indicated drugs may interact negatively with those the patient is using improperly; in other cases, the prescription of some classes of drugs may only contribute to the patient's drug problem (e.g., sedative-hypnotics, minor tranquilizers). Several licitly prescribed drugs are commonly abused: the nonbarbiturate depressants, diazepam (Valium), and chlordiazepoxide (Librium); sedative-hypnotics, barbiturates, methaqualone (Quaalude), and glutethimide (Doriden); stimulant-appetite suppressants (amphetamines and all other anorectics); and some analgesic drugs such as codeine, pentazocine (Talwin), and propoxyphene (Darvon).

A reasonably accurate assessment of the patient's rationality, along with the use of appropriate therapeutic measures (including psychotherapy or chemotherapy), should be included in the overall treatment plan that is developed for each patient. Most patients will require extensive social and economic guidance as part of the treatment plan. A variety of psychosocial rehabilitative services must often be provided, such as counseling, individual therapy, family therapy, and vocational, educational, or legal services. The failure rate increases if the patient returns to the drug-oriented peer environment from which he or she came.

Recognizing that each patient has unique dynamics, characteristics, and motivations is critical to effective treatment planning. The entire treatment staff, then, must know and understand as much as possible about each patient in order to deliver effective, high-quality care. Therefore, it is the responsibility of each member of the treatment team to obtain accurate information during the admission interview and each subsequent assessment. To do so demands that the physician and treatment team members remain as unbiased and nonjudgmental as possible during the interview process. Often, this means setting aside personal feelings, attitudes, and stereotypes about drug and alcohol abusers.

THE PERSONAL HISTORY INTERVIEW

During the personal history interview, the following areas should be covered: drug and alcohol history; social functioning; psychological functioning, including a review of such problems as disturbances in mood, suicide potential, impulse control, violence potential, conditioned response, and thought disorders; and sexual functioning.

Besides the specialized areas of history that should be elicited from the patient, a standard medical history should be taken that includes family history, individual history (with special emphasis being placed on medical problems frequently found in drug abusers), and a review of systems.

DRUG AND ALCOHOL HISTORY

To obtain complete information about the patient's drug and alcohol history, the physician must have information regarding the patient's age when alcohol or drugs were first used, the types and/or combinations of substances used, means of use (injected, taken orally, etc.), and numbers and types of previous treatments (if any).

When questioning the patient about his or her drug and alcohol history, it is essential that the physician approach the subject with sensitivity and discretion. Before direct questioning about drug and alcohol use, it is best to ask about the more socially acceptable drugs. The physician might first inquire about the frequency of the use of coffee and cigarettes; then about the use of any prescription drugs, including sedative-hypnotics, tranquilizers, antidepressants, etc.; proceeding to the use of wine, beer, and liquor; and finally on to illegally obtained drugs. Not only what drugs, but also why and what effect they provide, may give enlightening information.

Consideration of the drug or alcohol history is particularly important when dealing with a patient who tries to use the physician to obtain drugs. Frequently, such a patient will invent or exaggerate a medical problem in an effort to persuade the physician of the need for chemical relief. Simulation of the symptoms may be quite convincing; for example, acute renal colic may be simulated.

Nor is it unusual for a patient who is abusing drugs to be unaware of the problem. There are several common examples which should be kept in mind:

1. A person who uses amphetamines to lose weight and continues their use for a prolonged period develops a tolerance to the anorexigenic effect. Still, each time this person attempts to stop using the medication, something "doesn't feel right."
2. A chronic user of sleeping pills becomes tolerant to the hypnotic effect; yet if the patient fails to take the pills, he or she suffers from vivid nightmares, insomnia, and anxiety. The patient may even take the pills during the day in an attempt to reduce anxiety and depression.
3. Another example is the person who has become a chronic user of anxiolytics. (Diazepam, for instance, may lead to varying degrees of psychological and/or physical dependence, even at recommended daily dosages.)
4. Patients may begin to take an analgesic for general discomfort and nervousness, although the initial reason for the prescription was to combat chronic pain.
5. Analgesics (e.g., Darvon) may seem necessary to a patient's well-being because of withdrawal symptoms when the original need for an analgesic no longer exists.

There are also many patients who do not realize that drug or alcohol abuse is responsible for their medical problems. A patient with such complaints as pancreatitis, jaundice, and even insomnia may have a history of substance abuse which has generated these problems. This point cannot be stressed enough, and it is particularly crucial for those patients who are not aware of the relationship between the use of drugs and deteriorating health.

Whether the patient is consciously trying to manipulate the physician into prescribing drugs or is unconsciously trying to do so, it is important to keep in mind that persons who have had an alcohol abuse problem in the past are more likely than the average person to become habituated to drugs. The converse is also true—people who have been drug dependent in the past are more likely to become alcohol abusers or dependent on another drug.

SOCIAL FUNCTIONING

Assessments of current social functioning are made in almost all treatment programs as a matter of routine. They are practical, important, and provide essential information about the severity of the illness; they also provide an important baseline for evaluating treatment outcome. Social items often require outside corroboration, such as getting information from family or friends. In obtaining the outside corroborative material, the physician must remember not to violate the rules of confidentiality.

The physician or another member of the treatment staff should make inquiries into the patient's readiness for treatment, employment history, educational background, legal status, family life, social activities, and enrollment in other treatment programs. All of these factors are important elements of social functioning and should be noted. Urine test results can properly be recorded as an indicator of social functioning; they sometimes indicate what drugs the patient has been abusing.

When available, a vocational specialist should be included on the evaluation team to help determine whether or not vocational rehabilitation need be part of the treatment. Since medical factors may influence the type of vocational program that is selected, the physician should have a role in this aspect of the evaluation.

For specific questions that might be useful in collecting information in the above areas, see the Assessment Interviewing Guide (AIG), which appears in Appendix A. The AIG is an interview protocol designed to elicit information about the patient's lifestyle and life history. It contains more than 300 carefully phrased sample questions in four major content areas: Readiness for Treatment, Relationships, Rationality, and Resources.

PSYCHOLOGICAL FUNCTIONING

This subsection is intended to familiarize the physician with some of the ways to detect severe psychological disturbance. Although it is not necessary for the nonpsychiatrist physician to make a differential diagnosis, he or she should be able to determine that a psychiatric condition exists and refer the patient for further psychiatric evaluation.

A severe psychological disturbance is one important reason why patients fail in drug or alcohol abuse treatment. When patients do not respond in the usual way to treatment interventions, the possibility of a complicating underlying psychiatric condition should be considered. Presence of a severe psychological disturbance does not mean the patient is untreatable, but rather that the usual drug treatment plan must be modified to take the disturbance into account.

Effective treatment is now available for many types of psychological disturbance (e.g., depression and psychosis); if these problems are successfully treated through use of psychotherapy and/or psychotherapeutic drugs, the patient can frequently stay in a traditional alcohol or drug treatment program. Psychotherapeutic drugs should be used very cautiously with a drug abusing population, but they should be used when appropriate. Certain classes of psychotherapeutic drugs are rarely or never abused. Therapy can proceed as for other patients.

The physician should also be aware that psychological impairment can be an organic consequence of polydrug abuse. These abnormalities may show significant improvement if abstinence is maintained.

Drug and alcohol abuse may also complicate the treatment of a psychological disturbance. For example, changes in mood that are sufficiently extreme to warrant a diagnosis of manic-depressive illness are treatable with lithium. However, the patient's unreliable use of drugs or alcohol may make the use of lithium so hazardous that successful management in a routine drug treatment program is difficult; inpatient psychiatric treatment may be necessary.

Psychological Tests

Much effort has been expended in developing instruments that will help assess psychological and social functioning (written and projective tests), but few have stood the test of predictive validity with drug abusing patients. The Minnesota Multiphasic Personality Inventory

(MMPI) is the most popular of the tests being used, and despite the limitations associated with its use, its ease of administration and the availability of computerized scoring make periodic testing with the MMPI practical and useful in following a patient's progress.

Shorter tests, such as the Gordon and Wonderlic tests, and a measure of mood, such as the Beck Depression Inventory, are valuable measurements. Clinical psychological scales such as the NIMH 35-item Symptom Rating Scale, or a similar scale such as the Zung (both are anxiety and depression scales), may be helpful in measuring pretreatment symptoms of anxiety, depression, and agitation. The quantitative measurement of such variables is difficult under the best of conditions, as can be seen from a review of the literature. For further information about standard personality and psychological tests, refer to the current *Mental Measurements Yearbook* (Buros, 1978).

Psychiatric Problems

Drug and alcohol abuse may be associated with psychiatric problems. Several broad categories of these problems are discussed below, and suggestions are given for the type of questions that should be asked during a diagnostic interview:

Disturbances in mood. The patient should be asked questions designed to identify the presence of severe mood swings, such as those that occur during manic-depressive illness or severe depression. Periods of extreme elation not associated with a drug experience may be as pathological as periods of deep depression. The presence of severe mood disturbances indicates the need for referral for further psychiatric evaluation and perhaps initiation of psychiatric treatment. Fortunately, the affective disturbances (both depression and mania) are treatable. In some cases affective disturbances may even be the underlying reason for the drug abuse.

The following questions may be asked to assess present and past mood disturbances. (Italicized questions are drawn from the Assessment Interviewing Guide [Appendix A].)

1. Either before you were using alcohol or drugs, or at times when you had not been using them, have there been periods lasting days or weeks when—
    a. You could go for days without sleep?

b. Everything seemed unusually rosy?
   c. You went on binges—eating, spending, sex, gambling?
2. Either before you were using alcohol or drugs, or at times when you had not been using them, were there periods when you—
   a. Lost your appetite—had dramatic changes in weight, up or down (related to dieting)?
   b. Lost your sex drive?
   c. Had feelings of hopelessness or helplessness?
   d. Lost your ability to concentrate?
   e. Lost your interest or pleasure in things you usually enjoy?
   f. Had a dramatic change in sleeping patterns—slept too much or too little?
   g. Felt extremely depressed over a period of days or weeks?

Anxiety is a common disturbance in substance abusers. Frequently, the patient will call it "bad nerves," "tension," or "hypertension." The physician should inquire about the presence of anxiety and determine if alcohol or drugs relieve or exacerbate the problem. Specific drugs may have different effects on the anxiety; therefore, it is important to question the patient on how the anxiety responds to different drugs.

Suicide potential. The assessment of suicide potential is important not only to determine the immediate risk of suicide, but also to assess the patient's potential for harming himself or herself if loss, rage, or other strong negative affect occurs during treatment.

Sometimes the physician avoids discussing suicide for fear that it may plant the idea in the patient's mind. Generally speaking, this concern may be dimissed; most suicidal persons are relieved when the subject is broached directly.

The physician should ask the following questions:

1. *Have you ever had thoughts of harming yourself?*

2. *Have you ever had thoughts of killing yourself?*

3. *Have you ever feared that you might act on these thoughts?*

4. *Do you have these fears now or have you had them recently?*

5. *Have you ever attempted suicide?*

In assessing a patient's potential for suicide, the physician should inquire into other areas that often precipitate thoughts of suicide.

1. Does the patient live alone? Does he or she have any close friends or relatives?
2. Has the patient lost a close friend or relative recently?
3. Does the patient have a chronic illness? Is he or she caring for someone with a chronic illness?
4. Is there a history of suicide in the family?

Impulse control. Impulse control is the ability to avoid acting irrationally or inappropriately on strong thoughts or feelings. Evaluation of impulse control is of great prognostic importance in judging the patient's potential for completing treatment successfully. The patient with poor impulse control may get angry, quit the program, or act out according to his or her past lifestyle. The patient with good impulse control is more likely to continue in treatment and to behave in a predictable way.

Patients who can control their impulses in one area can learn to control them in others. Interview questions, therefore, should tap a range of experiences in which impulse control plays a role.

The physician should ask the following questions:

1. *Can you wait for something or must you have it now?*
2. *If you drive, how many miles did you drive last year?*
3. *How many times were you stopped for a moving violation?*
4. *Have you ever been on a diet and been able to stick to it?*
5. *How do you handle your anger?*
6. *How will I know when you get angry at me?*
7. *How do you handle frustration?*
8. *How do you handle money?*
9. *Do you budget?*
10. *Can you save money?*
11. *If you have a 3-day supply of dope, can you spread it out and make it last 3 days?*

Violence potential. The patient's potential for violence, if high, may be a severe limitation both in terms of referral and in treatment management. Patients may be violent in one of two ways. Some may display impulsive violence when angry or frustrated; this type of violence is largely unpredictable and can disrupt the clinic or ward. Assessment of impulsive violence potential is interrelated with the assessment of impulse control. Other patients are violent but have good impulse control; they can plan acts in advance (such as armed robbery) and carry them out successfully.

Because differentiation between the two forms of violence is based primarily on the individual's history, the circumstances surrounding episodes of violent behavior should be explored in detail. Comprehensive assessment includes global evaluation of the patient's lifestyle, impulse control, and coping styles. The existence of an arrest record, by itself, cannot be equated with violence potential. For example, the person apprehended for armed robbery most likely has a higher potential for violence than one apprehended for drug possession. Individuals who commit crimes against property, such as writing bad checks, or victimless crimes, such as prostitution, usually have a lower violence potential.

Some patients may be violent only when intoxicated. This violence is related to the poor judgment and diminished impulse control that frequently accompanies intoxication and is generally a better prognostic sign than is impulsive violence while not using drugs or drinking heavily. The physician should ask the patient the following questions:

1. *Have you ever harmed anyone?* (If yes) *Who was it? What were the circumstances?*

2. *Were you under the influence of drugs or alcohol at that time?*

3. *Was it survival or self-defense?*

4. *Was it revenge?*

NOTE: Take into consideration data from the patient's arrest record, if he or she has one.

For other methods of determining possible psychological disturbances, see Table 3-1, Checklist: A Summary of the Interview Behavior.

If aberrant behavior is noted, it may indicate intoxication, underlying emotional disturbance, or a personality trait.

Conditioned responses. The patient's conditioned responses to drug-related stimuli are a psychological indicator that has frequently

Table 3-1
CHECKLIST: A SUMMARY OF THE INTERVIEW BEHAVIOR

Yes	No	
		Behavior:
___	___	Friendly
___	___	Intoxicated
___	___	Hyperactive
___	___	Inactive
___	___	Alert
___	___	Initiates conversation
___	___	Nervous
___	___	Manipulative
___	___	Seductive
___	___	Directs the interview
___	___	Evasive
___	___	Suspicious
___	___	Believable
___	___	Cooperative
___	___	Behavior appropriate to interview situation
		Thought disorder:
___	___	Does the patient make sense?
___	___	Is he thinking straight?
___	___	Can you follow him?
___	___	Does his attention wander?
___	___	Does he answer questions appropriately?
___	___	Is the patient scared?
___	___	Does he scare you?
		Sensorium orientation:
		Is the patient oriented to
___	___	Time?
___	___	Place?
___	___	Person?
___	___	Situation?

been neglected in the evaluation of drug dependence. These conditioned responses are another measure of the drug abuser's degree of addiction. If, for example, a patient develops withdrawal or craving responses when he or she enters a specific environment, the treatment procedure might include efforts to help the patient avoid that environment, or, if that is not possible, to decondition these responses through behavior modification techniques. If a patient gets a high from the process of self-injecting (a so-called "needle freak"), appropriate therapy should be designed to decondition this behavior. The strength of such responses may be measured by determining the frequency of the responses and the exact conditions under which they occur. This measure may show initial severity of dependence, and also may be one that could be monitored throughout treatment to determine progress. Although work on such technology is still experimental, the existence of conditioned responses should be kept in mind during evaluation because of its implications for therapy.

Thought disorders. Thought disorders (which may be a manifestation of psychosis) are clinically defined as a flow of thought that may become seemingly haphazard, purposeless, illogical, apparently confused, abrupt, and bizarre. Thought disorders are most frequently found in schizophrenia, toxic reactions, and organic brain damage. Thought disorders may be characterized by the following:

1. *Disturbances in the form of thinking* includes all deviations from rational, logical, goal-directed thinking. In this type of thinking, the facts of reality are not considered. Hallucinations and delusions are the most common symptoms.
   a. *Hallucination* is an apparent perception of an external object when no corresponding external object exists. It can be auditory, visual, tactile, gustatory, or olfactory.
   b. *Delusion* is a false belief that arises in the face of contrary evidence without appropriate personal or culturally determined knowledge.
2. *Disturbances in stream of thought* are abnormalities in the manner and rate of the associations made in thinking. Some of the most common symptoms are listed below:
   a. *Blocking* is a sudden stop in the flow of thought or speech in the middle of a sentence. The person is usually unable to continue the sentence, and when he or she tries, a new idea crops up unconnected to the original thought.
   b. *Intellectualization* is a state of brooding or anxious pondering about abstract, theoretical, or philosophical issues. The concepts are usually emotionally neutral.
   c. *Circumstantiality* is the verbalization of too many associated ideas. Excessive detail is used to describe simple events, at

times to an absurd or bizarre degree. The goal of the thought is eventually reached after many digressions. Extreme forms occur in schizophrenia and organic brain disease.

d. *Tangential thinking* means that the goal of the thought is never reached, and the thought is not on target.

e. *Perseveration* is the tendency for an act of behavior, an attitude, or mental or physical set to persist or remount into consciousness spontaneously after it has once occurred and is no longer appropriate to the situation at hand.

f. *Incoherence* is the result of disorderly thinking; i.e., thoughts do not follow in a logical sequence in such a way that verbalizations can be understood by the listener.

g. *Flight of ideas* is characterized by a nearly continuous, high-speed flow of speech, jumping from one topic to another, with an illogical progression of thought. It is characteristic of manic states.

h. *Aphasia* is any language problem resulting from organic brain damage in which the defect is not due to faulty innervation of speech musculature or general mental deficiency. The language problem is due to poor comprehension, symbolization, and reproduction of concepts during speech or writing.

3. *Disturbances in content of thought* are characterized by the patient's emphasizing that his or her thoughts are inexpressible.

   Obsession is the pathological presence of a persistent and irresistible thought, feeling, or impulse that cannot be eliminated by logical effort.

4. *Disturbances of orientation* occur when the patient is unable to recognize him or herself in his surroundings and to comprehend their relationship to time and space. Orientation to time (year, month, day of month, day of week), person, and place is called *sensorium*. Other characteristics in this category include recent and remote memory, *retention,* and *immediate recall*. Impaired sensorium is found most commonly in organic brain disease.

5. *Disturbances in judgment* are similar in manifestation to poor impulse control and a fairly high potential for violence (discussed previously). Judgment is the mental act of comparing or evaluating alternatives within the framework of a given set of values and considering the possible consequences connected with the alternatives for the purpose of deciding on a course of action. The controlled postponement or elimination of action,

then, is the essence of judgment. In the context of the mainstream of social values, most drug or alcohol abusers can be said to have exercised *poor* judgment. In the clinical sense, pathological disturbance of judgment is present when a patient continually and consistently avoids confronting reality by choosing alternatives he or she feels will be less painful. These alternatives may appear to be more immediately rewarding, but in the long run, they may be counterproductive or even self-destructive.

In summary, confusion of thought in general, and thought disorders in particular, may indicate severe mental disturbances; caution must be exercised in assessing disorders of this type. Some of the symptoms described above can result from drug and alcohol abuse per se, and some can be found in a patient who is intoxicated. Vast cultural differences may give the physician an impression of thought disorder when, in fact, the problem is one of communication style and verbal facility. Problems of expression may be intensified if the patient is highly emotional. When the possibility for this problem exists, a consulting physician who is closer to the patient's cultural background should be asked to interview the patient. The symptoms in such cases may not be indicative of a serious underlying psychopathology.

When interviewing the drug or alcohol dependent person the interviewer must always be aware that the patient may be giving false information. This may be part of the "conning" behavior that is so important for "street" survival. Because this behavior is not uncommon, the interviewer should try to verify all information by asking the same type of question several times during the interview to see if the client is consistent, and the physician should also seek verification from other sources. When a second source is used, confidentiality must be maintained.

In addition to the patient's responses to questions, observation of the behavior during the interview situation provides important information. The Checklist Summary of the Interview Behavior (Table 3-1) is designed to be completed *after* the assessment interview. It is an example of one way in which observations may be recorded quickly and concisely on a checklist. The main purpose of this inventory is to help identify patients who may have psychological disturbances that would not be evidenced by direct questioning. Some treatment programs may wish to modify or adapt the inventory to suit their own special purposes.

SEXUAL FUNCTIONING

Inadequate sexual functioning may be a major problem for the patient applying for treatment. Substance abuse may contribute to a patient's sexual dysfunction. A detailed sexual history (assessing development and current status) should therefore be conducted, preferably before or early on in treatment by the physician or a member of the staff. The initial discussion should be brief, because the patient may consider it an intrusion of privacy.

After some rapport has been established between patient and physician, a complete history of the patient's sexual functioning should be completed. The current level of sexual functioning must be assessed so that the effects of treatment on this area can be evaluated. Drugs and alcohol can have a marked effect on sexual functioning. Opiates decrease libido and may initially depress pituitary sex hormones until tolerance develops. Males complain of delayed ejaculation during high-dose use of opiates. On the other hand, spontaneous ejaculations occur during withdrawal or with irregular use of opiates. In women, the depression of hormonal function may result in amenorrhea or irregular menstrual cycles and may decrease fertility. Methadone has similar effects on sexual functions, as do other opiates. However, when methadone is used in maintenance doses, the primary complaints are decreased libido and delayed ejaculation. Some patients on methadone maintenance feel the delayed ejaculation is a positive effect since they are able to prolong intercourse.

The chronic use of depressant drugs (including alcohol) in high doses may result in the person's inability to have an erection or orgasm. Potency usually returns to normal when the use stops. Stimulant drugs usually increase sexual desires but also delay ejaculation or orgasm. Alcohol and opiates lower testosterone levels both by actions on the testes and by alterations of hepatic function. Marijuana has been reported to lower testosterone levels and diminish sperm counts, but this alteration has not been found consistently by all investigations. The significance of these findings has not been fully evaluated.

If substance abuse begins during adolescence when development of sexual functioning is occurring and feelings of inadequacy are common, the use of drugs may be an attempt to repair the user's damaged self-esteem. Thus, inadequate sexual functioning may be either the cause or the effect of drug abuse.

Some drug or alcohol abusers have never had sexual relations except when intoxicated. This possibility should be ascertained, since extensive counseling may be required before sexual relations are satisfactorily resumed during treatment. The physician should remember that sexual problems may not be reported by the patient unless specific questions are asked, but that the diagnosis of sexual problems is essential to adequate treatment.

REFERENCES

Buros, O. K. (ed.) *The eighth mental measurements yearbook.* Highland Park, New Jersey: Gryphon Press, 1978.

Jones G. H. The recognition of alcoholism by psychiatrists in training. *Psychological Medicine,* 1979, *9,* 789-791.

4
The Physical Examination

A thorough physical examination should be performed following the procedures outlined in many standard references on diagnosis. During the physical examination, the physician should be aware of some of the more common signs and symptoms of drug abuse.

SIGNS AND SYMPTOMS OF DRUG AND ALCOHOL ABUSE

The patient's presenting medical problem may be caused by substance abuse, or it may be totally independent of it. Drug and alcohol abusers may become severely debilitated; consequently, debilitation that does not result from the medical problems overtly presented should raise the suspicion of substance abuse. This possibility should be considered if abnormalities appear in the patient's speech and movement patterns, pupils or skin (abscesses, edema), or in the case of ulcerations in the nasal mucosa, multiple traumas from accidents, or pressure palsies of peripheral nerves from deep, intoxicated sleep.

The physician should be particularly alert to the possible medical complications that are either directly or indirectly related to drug and alcohol abuse. Hence, in the initial stages of the physical examination, the physician should look for the cutaneous signs of drug abuse, which can be readily divided into two categories of sequelae: direct and indirect. (See Table 4-1.)

DIRECT SEQUELAE

Listed below are direct sequelae:

1. Skin tracks and related scars are the most important direct cutaneous signs of drug abuse. These result from intravenous injections and occur on the neck, axilla, forearm, wrist, hand, foot,

Table 4-1
CUTANEOUS SIGNS OF ALCOHOL AND DRUG ABUSE

Direct Sequelae		Indirect Sequelae	
Local	**Systematic**	**Other Stigmata**	**Medical Problems**
Skin tracks	Fixed drug eruption	Excoriations	Jaundice
Pop scars	Eyelid edema	Acne excoriée	Pigmentary problems
Abscess	Urticaria	Self-induced tattoos	Pseudo-acanthosis nigricans
Ulceration	Purpura	Wrist scars	Bullous impetigo
Infection	Pruritus	Tourniquet pigmentation	Cheilitis
Sphaceloderma		Perianal solvent rash	Contact dermatitis
Hand edema			Cigarette burns
Thrombophlebitis			Dental disorders
Camptodactyly			
Shooting tattoo			
Bullae			
Perforated septum			
Acne rosacea			
Spider nevi			
Palmar erythema			
Porphyria cutanea tarda			

ankle, under the tongue, and on the dorsal vein of the penis. The marks are usually multiple, hyperpigmented, and linear. New lesions may be inflamed. The scars may fade slowly over the course of a year or more, or may never fade. (Skin tracks are discussed in more detail elsewhere.)
2. Needle puncture marks are usually located over veins and may be indicative of recent injection. Such marks usually disappear within a week.
3. Pop scars from skin popping (subcutaneous drug injections), are found on the arm, especially in the deltoid and gluteal areas, abdomen, thigh, and scapula. These scars are permanent circumscribed depressions in the skin similar to pock marks.
4. Abscesses, infection, and ulceration are infective and chemical reactions to the injections. They are seen on the arm, thigh, shoulder, abdomen, chest, hand, and finger.
5. Gangrene of the skin (sphaceloderma) has been seen in drug abusers.
6. Hand edema and irreducible finger flexion (camptodactyly) are found in abusers who inject into finger or hand veins.
7. Thrombophlebitis often occurs at the site of the injection.
8. Accidental tattoos due to carbon from flaming a needle are often seen at the injection site; these will slowly disappear.
9. Bullae may appear owing to hot solutions injected under the skin or to barbiturate overdose.
10. A toxic dermatitis, called fixed drug eruption, can occur at the injection site.
11. Both purpura and urticaria, probably due to allergic reactions, are found in abusers, as is pruritis.
12. Snorting heroin or cocaine can cause ulcerations or even perforation of the nasal septum of the drug abuser from irritation and infection of the nasal mucosa.
13. Chronic alcohol abusers may have acne rosacea (dilation of vessels on the nose) with thickening of the skin, spider nevi (dilated subcutaneous arterioles over the upper third of the body area with blanching on pressure), palmar erythema, and porphyria cutanea tarda with blistering and erythema.

INDIRECT SEQUELAE

The following are indirect sequelae:

1. Both self-induced excoriations from itching and acne excoriée are common.
2. Tattoos of figures, characters, and words related to drug abuse, indicative of the need to belong to a group, are seen. Tattoos may be placed to cover tracks.
3. Wrist scars are seen on abusers who have attempted suicide by slashing their wrists. Depression and suicide attempts frequently occur among drug and alcohol abusers.
4. Tourniquet pigmentation is a poorly defined linear mark that appears above the antecubital space from the repeated use of cord-like or belt-like materials as tourniquets for intravenous injections.
5. Jaundice is a common physical sign arising from hepatitis-shared equipment.
6. Sometimes either hypopigmentation or hyperpigmentation develops in the drug abuser, specifically in the areas around injection.
7. Pseudo-acanthosis nigricans is sometimes seen in the axillae of the drug abuser; the cause is unknown.
8. Bullous impetigo (staphylococcal) is sometimes found in long-time drug abusers.
9. Cheilitis (cracking of skin at corners of mouth) can frequently be seen during or prior to detoxification and is possibly related to dehydration or hypovitaminosis.
10. Contact dermatitis can result from sensitivity to the antiseptics to prepare the skin before injection. It is also seen around the nose, mouth, and hands of solvent users, in which case it is known as "glue-sniffer's rash."
11. Cigarette burns due to drowsiness are sometimes found, especially between the fingers and on the chest.
12. Dental disorders, usually caused by neglect and poor nutrition, are not uncommon in drug abusers.
13. Trench mouth may also be found in drug abusers, secondary to poor oral hygiene.
14. Skin infections and infestations are usually secondary to poor

hygiene and may be caused by scabies, lice, fungi, and bacteria.
15. Piloerection (gooseflesh) is seen in withdrawal from opiates and appears primarily on the trunk and arms.

5
Diagnosis of Medical Complications of Alcohol and Drug Abuse

MEDICAL COMPLICATIONS OF ALCOHOL AND DRUG ABUSE

The following discussion focuses on the most common medical complications of drug abuse.

DERMATOLOGICAL COMPLICATIONS

Most complications of drug abuse come not from the drug itself, but from the conditions under which it is taken. Infectious complications are due to unsterile and contaminated injections. The source of the organisms is most commonly the skin and nasopharynx, although other areas of the body may be the cause for contamination. However, the drug mixture with its adulterants, the diluent, and the injection paraphernalia may also be sources of viruses, bacteria, or fungi.

Septic Cutaneous Complications

The following septic cutaneous complications are discussed first because the skin is the port of entry of contaminated injections:

1. Needle-track scars are caused by unsterile techniques and the injection of fibrogenic particulate matter.
2. In addition, attempts to sterilize the needle by heating the tip

with a match causes carbon to be deposited on it, which causes mild inflammatory reaction. Subsequent repeated injection with such a needle causes tattooing or dark pigmentation at the point of entry of the needle. However, macrophages pick up the carbon, and the tracks become progressively lighter.

Although most common on the arms, tracks can be found on almost any part of the body, because abusers realize that the arms are the first area to be checked. Even the penile veins have been used for injection. The subcutaneous scars found on the thighs and arms are due to chronic abscesses.

3. Abscess formation (the most common septic problem) is usually easy to recognize. Repeated injections without cleansing the skin around the injection sites produce infections that are most commonly due to skin flora, i.e., staphylococci and streptococci. Anaerobic infections, however, occur at a much higher rate in the drug user who takes the drug parenterally. These abscesses may sometimes be recognized by the presence of a foul-smelling discharge, less often by gas formation, and by a bizarre type of cellulitis.
4. This cellulitis (perhaps really a fasciolitis) is characterized by a stony or wooden-hard tenseness, which progresses rapidly on an extremity, and not necessarily in association with a recent needle puncture or infected site. Cellulitis occurs when sedative-hypnotics are injected subcutaneously. The tissue becomes reddened, hot, painful, and swollen.
5. Another complication in an extremity may be caused by intraarterial injection. Intense pain is usually produced distal to the site of injection. Swelling, cyanosis, and coldness of the extremity indicate the onset of a medical emergency. If untreated, gangrene of the hands or fingers may develop with consequent loss of these parts (sphaceloderma).
6. Camptodactyly results from recurrent use of the hand veins for injection. Irreversible contracture of the fingers and lymphedema may result.

Pruritus and Dermatitis

Pruritis alone, or in combination with urticaria, may be seen in heroin abusers. Contact dermatitis results from sensitization to exotic fluids used to sterilize the skin.

SPECIFIC INFECTIONS

Tetanus

Tetanus is a problem seen today almost exclusively in heroin abusers. Since 1955, 70% to 90% of reported tetanus cases have occurred in drug abusers. Its mortality rate approaches 90%.

Heroin abusers with tetanus are usually female (a 3:1 ratio). This results because skin popping is more common in women, who generally have poorer venous development than men, which makes intravenous injection more difficult. Moreover, women are less frequently immunized against tetanus. By injecting into the subcutaneous fat where there is poor vascularization, there is an increased chance that anaerobic infection will develop.

The limitation of tetanus to the East Coast and Chicago results from the inclusion of 2% to 10% quinine in the drug mixture in these areas. Quinine is a protoplasmic poison that reduces the redox potential, thus providing perfect conditions on intramuscular injection for the germination of Clostridium tetani. Because dogs act as carriers of the organism, it is widespread.

Malaria

Malaria, another complication of drug abuse, is closely associated with mainlining. It was first reported in New Orleans in drug-abusing, needle-sharing sailors who had been exposed to malaria in Africa.

When infected World War II veterans returned, malaria was seen in New York, but disappeared in that city in the late 1940's. It hasn't been seen there since, probably because of quinine in the drug mixture in that area. Although the daily dose of quinine in the mixture won't eradicate the disease, quinine is such a severe protoplasmic poison that it presumably kills the malarial parasites in the syringe.

With the return of veterans from Vietnam, there was an increase in drug-related malaria, but this took place solely on the West Coast, where quinine was not being used in the drug mixtures.

CARDIOVASCULAR COMPLICATIONS

Endocarditis

Endocarditis has attracted more attention than the other complications of drug abuse. The exact magnitude of this problem is difficult to determine because many drug abusers with cardiovascular complications die outside the hospital or have such short hospital stays that no diagnosis is made.

The most important cardiovascular complication of drug abuse is acute infective endocarditis. In order of frequency, the valves most commonly affected are the aortic, mitral, and tricuspid. Recent reports have described a few cases of pulmonic valve endocarditis that mimic tricuspid endocarditis. Although right-sided endocarditis in a drug abuser is frequent, left-sided endocarditis occurs twice as often. In addition, a significant number (5% to 10%) of abusers have both right- and left-sided (mixed) lesions.

Among heroin abusers there is a high frequency of staphylococcal, gram-negative bacterial and candidal valve infections, while streptococcal infections are practically nonexistent. Preexisting heart disease is less frequently found in the heroin abusing population developing endocarditis than in the nondrug-abusing population that develops endocarditis.

The unusually high incidence of endocarditis occurring in normal valves in heroin abusers is probably due to the repetitive bacteremias and the virulence of the organisms isolated, especially coagulase-positive Staphylococcus aureus. The higher incidence of endocarditis due to Candida and to gram-negative bacilli in heroin abusers with endocarditis results from unsterilized equipment and unusual methods of injection. Candida infections, which affect damaged valves, occur less frequently in abusers with right-sided involvement. Recently, Pseudomonas has been isolated in patients with tricuspid endocarditis.

Infective endocarditis should be suspected in any drug abuser who presents with fever of unknown origin, heart murmur, pneumonia, embolic phenomena, or positive blood cultures (especially with Candida, Staphylococcus aureus, enterococci, or gram-negative organisms). Fever may be the only indication of endocarditis, even with negative cultures.

Because endocarditis in abusers is often fulminating, usually producing the frequent embolization and severe valve destruction of acute endocarditis, it is imperative that this condition be suspected and treatment begun early if the patient is to survive.

Although septic pulmonary emboli may develop in abusers following thrombophlebitis with endocarditis, and because tricuspid involvement may occur without heart murmur, it is advisable to assume that patients with septic pulmonary emboli have endocarditis.

Abusers being treated for staphylococcal pneumonia (and acute meningitis) should be observed for 7 to 10 days after completion of therapy with antibiotics to avoid overlooking the early signs and symptoms of endocarditis.

Pneumococcal endocarditis is the most common endocardial complication among chronic alcoholics. Pneumococcal meningitis is also very common.

Other Cardiovascular Complications

Infective endocarditis is the most destructive cardiovascular complication. Other cardiac problems include myocardial disease (possibly due to direct toxic effects of some drugs on the myocardium), blood pressure changes, and cardiac arrhythmias. Vascular complications include local changes due to thrombophlebitis, arteritis, arterial occlusion, embolic phenomena, angio-thrombotic pulmonary hypertension, and other problems due to traumatic or mycotic aneurysms.

Alcoholic cardiomyopathy is the result of the direct toxic effect of alcohol or its metabolite, acetaldehyde. Beriberi heart disease is a rare complication of thiamine deficiency in malnourished alcoholics. Beer drinker's heart consists of right-handed failure, hypertension, and pericardial effusion. It has been attributed to cobalt, but lead contamination is also a possibility.

Tachyarrythmias occur with many drugs of abuse. Cannabis, cocaine, hallucinogens, amphetamines, and anticholinergic drugs accelerate the pulse rate.

Vascular changes due to necrotizing angiitis (polyarteritis) have been demonstrated in intravenous amphetamine abusers (mainly methamphetamine), resulting in cerebrovascular occlusion and intracranial hemorrhage. Many of the solvents used by "glue sniffers" cause a sensitization of the heart to catecholamines similar to that seen with volatile anesthetics. This reaction can lead to sudden death (if ventricular fibrillation occurs) or to arrhythmias. Also, tricyclic antidepressants, although not commonly considered drugs of abuse, have been increasingly abused in the past few years. In high doses, they can cause arrhythmias due to a direct irritant action on the myocardium. Phencyclidine, cocaine, and amphetamines can produce paroxysmal hypertension. In high doses, the hypertension must be treated vigorously.

PULMONARY COMPLICATIONS

Because the lung is the primary filtering organ of insoluble material administered intravenously, insoluble particulate materials that are used to adulterate I.V.-administered drugs lodge in the lung; this causes multiple microinfarcts. The most common cutting agents are talc, starch, lactose, and bicarbonate of soda. Talc, being the most insoluble of these materials, is the agent that most frequently causes the microinfarcts. Long-term intravenous self-administration of drugs such as amphetamines and methylphenidate (Ritalin) leads to this type of complication. Because amphetamines most commonly come in tablet form for oral use, intravenous use results in the depositing of large amounts of insoluble fillers in the lungs, in the same way that the insoluble substances in heroin are deposited. This insoluble matter in the pulmonary vasculature produces chronic pulmonary fibrosis and foreign-body granulomas, resulting in poor oxygen diffusion across the alveolar capillary membranes. This leads to resulting changes in lung elasticity. The pulmonary hypertension produced may cause cardiac failure. Chest X-rays may be normal or show bilateral fine reticular basilar infiltrates, pulmonary artery enlargement, or hilar adenopathy. Pulmonary hypertension has also been reported following high-dose oral amphetamine abuse. This is probably due to a direct effect of amphetamine on the pulmonary vasculature.

Intravenous administration of illicit drugs can also cause pulmonary parenchymal contamination with a large number of bacteria. These bacteria may come from the drug itself, the diluents, the paraphernalia, or from the body of the abuser. Whatever the source, this contamination can cause pulmonary infections with bacteria not normally isolated in pneumonitis. Pulmonary abscesses can also be due to infections of the heart valves, particularly the tricuspid and pulmonic valves. The constant seeding of such bacteria into the pulmonary circulation results in intrapulmonary infections that are difficult to manage.

The most serious pulmonary effect of drug abuse is probably that associated with depressant and heroin overdose, which severely depresses the respiratory center, resulting in apnea and death from anoxia. Acute pulmonary edema has also been noted frequently in opiate overdose. Pulmonary edema, in combination with the depression of the respiratory center as seen with narcotic overdose, often brings about death unless appropriate treatment is initiated. This type of pulmonary edema can also be produced by propoxyphene (Darvon) and methadone overdoses.

Aspiration pneumonia must be clinically differentiated from pulmonary edema in heroin overdose patients. Drug abusers are frequently dropped off at an emergency room after unsuccessful attempts at revival with large quantities of milk, coffee, Coca-Cola, or other substances. These ineffective efforts to manage the overdose usually do little more than cause the person to aspirate these substances. Pulmonary edema from overdose may have an associated fever of up to 101 degrees and a leukocytosis of 25,000 to 30,000. Both generally return to normal within 48 hours. Because of the importance of early steroid therapy in treating aspiration pneumonia, a helpful differential point is the presence of slowed or normal respirations in pulmonary edema (secondary to depression of the respiratory center), as opposed to increased respirations in aspiration pneumonia.

Chronic drug abuse may be extremely debilitating—lung infections frequently arise. Opiates depress the cough reflex. In the stuporous and debilitated abuser who may be vomiting, aspiration pneumonia frequently results. This has been observed with all forms of depressant drugs, and the resulting pneumonias often involve bacteria that are difficult to deal with. Debilitation may also lead to tuberculosis in the drug abuser.

Chronic uvulitis, pharyngitis, and bronchitis have been reported in heavy smokers. Bronchitis is associated with cocaine freebase.

Tuberculosis and pneumonia are found among malnourished alcoholics whose lifestyle includes poor hygiene and overcrowding. Reduced immune response also plays a role.

HEPATIC COMPLICATIONS

Hepatitis is the most common medical complication of drug abuse. In some hospitals, as many as 90% of admissions for hepatitis results from parenteral drug abuse infections. One study of heroin abusers revealed that fewer than 10% of abusers who took their heroin by insufflation (snorting) showed SGOT levels greater than 250 (almost 60% had normal levels). In abusers who used the needle even as seldom as once, more than 35% had levels of 250 or more, with 66% showing the presence of some liver disease. Of heroin abusers who had had hepatitis, 80% reported that the problem developed within 2 years after the first needle use.

The Australia antigen has become the prime means of detecting serum hepatitis (hepatitis B, long-incubation hepatitis) in drug abusers. This antigen is present in 50% to 70% of abusers with overt hepatitis. In a normal population, the incidence of positive readings is 0.1% to 0.2%; among heroin abusers, it is 2% to 8%. The frequency of a positive Australia antigen in needle users has been reported to be as high as 22.4% in some series. These figures indicate the public health problem resulting from the increased incidence of hepatitis in recipients of transfusions of blood obtained from drug abusing donors and in medical personnel who accidentally prick their skin with needles or glassware contaminated by the blood of drug abusers having hepatitis.

Although serum hepatitis was formerly thought to be transmitted only by entry of the virus through broken skin (by contaminated needle or transfusion of blood from a carrier), it is now known that this virus can be transmitted by biting insects (mosquitoes), oral intake of the infectious agent, and perhaps through sexual intercourse.

Pathological changes in the livers of drug abusers are common. Some of the histological changes include acute hepatitis, fibrosis or chronic active disease, and focal inflammation. The histological findings of acute liver disease in drug abusers may be more dramatic than the disease itself; indeed, compared to nonabusers with similar histological changes, the prognosis is better. So-called "junk" hepatitis, possibly the result of the contaminated material brought into the vein along with the drug, is characterized histologically by a more significant infiltration and inflammation of the portal tract, where eosinophils and various other inflammatory cells may be seen. This form of hepatitis seems to be a histological manifestation only, and has little effect on the outcome of the disease.

Chronic liver disease is a major problem in patients who have liver abnormalities secondary to drug abuse. Among persons with acute reversible hepatitis, the incidence of drug abuse is about 60%; with chronic persistent or chronic progressive hepatitis, the incidence of drug abuse is 80%; and with postnecrotic cirrhosis associated with viral hepatitis, the incidence of drug abuse is 90%.

Australia antigen-positive drug abusers thus have a very high incidence of chronicity, characterized by fibrosis or chronic progressive hepatitis.

Antigen-negative drug abusers who may have been positive earlier also have some incidence of chronicity; the same is true of 15% to 20% of those who are antigen-positive who have sporadic or multiple episodes of hepatitis.

Alcoholism alone or alcoholism and drug abuse together may lead to cirrhosis. In fact, the drug abuser with hepatitis is three to four times more likely to have hepatic fibrosis if he drinks more than 32 ounces of alcohol a week than the abuser who drinks less than 10 ounces a week.

Steatosis of the liver (fatty liver) is a reversible condition following upon an alcoholic bout. Recurrent, excessive drinking with or without nutritional insufficiency can result in chronic hepatitis. After a number of alcoholic exacerbations of hepatitis, cirrhosis may develop. Liver cirrhosis is the fourth leading cause of death among men over 40 years of age in some cities. The most sensitive test for alcoholic liver injury is the gamma glutamyltranspeptidase (GGT) test.

Although hepatic carcinoma is rare, it has occurred in Australia antigen-positive patients and may eventually prove to have a higher incidence in substance abusers. Physicians must be alert to this possibility so that its diagnosis and treatment is accurate and early.

Liver necrosis has been reported as a complication of solvent abuse. Recent evidence, however, indicates that this is not a problem with intermittent low-dose users but is found to be associated with chronic exposure such as may occur in industrial settings. Workers exposed in industrial settings will often take solvents home to continue the exposure after working hours.

REPRODUCTIVE SYSTEM COMPLICATIONS

Drug abusers have a higher than average incidence of gonorrhea, syphilis, chancroid, and lymphogranuloma venerum. Narcotic addicts have high rates of both true and false positive serological reactions for syphilis. A biological false positive is found in about 25% of all positives.

Chronic use of the CNS depressants eventually impairs potency and libido. With alcohol and other depressants, decreased testosterone levels may be found. Stimulants, cannabis, and the volatile nitrites have been used to maintain erection, prolong orgasm, or intensify the subjective sexual experience.

Although women who abuse drugs frequently have irregular menses, either from the action of the drug or nutritional factors, the most important diagnostic finding with respect to the reproductive system in a drug abusing patient (apart from specific sexual dysfunction) is the determination of whether a patient is pregnant. Estimates suggest that some 80% of drug dependent women are of childbearing age (14-40), which suggests a significant likelihood of pregnancy among women coming for treatment.

Although menstrual dysfunction frequently accompanies drug abuse—particularly heroin abuse—drug dependent women can become pregnant. Cessation of menstruation and other irregularities appear less frequently in the methadone-maintained patient. If the chief symptom of pregnancy—a change in menstruation—is missing, it may be difficult for the woman to realize that she is pregnant. Indications are that the number of live births among dependent women is increasing, even though rates of spontaneous abortion and illegal abortion are also high.

The determination of pregnancy is an important part of diagnosis and evaluation for two reasons. First, as is true for any female patient, every effort should be made to ensure adequate prenatal and postnatal care. Since the drug abusing woman is less likely than the average pregnant patient to seek care, the opportunity for the physician to influence such care is significant. Second, pregnancy in a drug abuser is an important consideration in the design of a treatment plan. Although some have recommended complete withdrawal from drugs during pregnancy, there are significant dangers to the fetus if withdrawal occurs—particularly in the latter stages of pregnancy. Any decision to attempt to withdraw a pregnant patient should be made by comparing the risks of withdrawal with the risks of continued maintenance drug use. The usual treatment is to switch the mother to a drug such as low doses of methadone, thereby removing the complications of street drug use. Although drugs like methadone easily pass through the placenta to the fetus, and the possibility of creating methadone dependence in the fetus exists, this is usually less of a medical risk than continued illicit drug use or sudden withdrawal.

An opiate dependent mother converted to methadone is usually maintained on a low dosage (less than 40 mg). Gradual withdrawal from methadone can be accomplished under close medical supervision without causing great difficulty to mother or fetus.

Federal methadone regulations require informed consent by the female patient of child bearing age to the use of methadone. The patient must be informed that methadone will cause physical dependence in an unborn child and that scientific knowledge as to its effects is inadequate to guarantee that it will not produce serious side effects.

It should be noted here that research with respect to sexuality and sexual functioning in the female drug abuser is more limited than it is for men.

NEUROMUSCULAR COMPLICATIONS

The exact etiologic factor in the (rare) neurological complications of drug abuse are difficult to evaluate because of the complexity of the crude, unsterile mixtures taken and the methods of administration. For example, transverse myelitis, plexitis, and acute rhabdomyolysis may arise after a period of abstinence from heroin, or they may be seen following a single injection after a drug-free period.

The discovery of immunoglobulin and complement in the kidneys of heroin abusers who develop nephrotic syndrome may implicate heroin abuse as an infectious, toxic, or immunologic stimulus that may be expressed as a neuritis, vasculitis, or nephrotic syndrome. Alcoholic myopathy can occur early in heavy drinkers.

Noninfectious Neurological Complications

The heroin overdose without contamination, like overdoses with other opium alkaloids, is characterized by coma, depressed respiration, tachycardia, and contracted pupils. The overdose may be complicated, however, by convulsive seizures and increased intracranial pressure, which is often associated with pulmonary edema and which may be related to a hypersensitivity to the adulterants.

Convulsive seizures are usually of the grand mal type. Focal seizures and status epilepticus also occur, but the seizures usually stop at the time of recovery from the withdrawal without subsequent attacks.

Cerebral sequelae may occur after an overdose. After a severe overdose reaction, the patient may go through a period of acute delirium with agitation, tremors, and hallucinosis lasting several hours to several days. In rare cases, the delirium may be the forerunner of chronic organic brain dysfunction, probably resulting from anoxia due to the overdose.

Cardiorespiratory arrest following overdose may be accompanied by delayed, postanoxic encephalopathy.

Although not common, cerebrovascular accidents with embolic phenomena may follow heroin overdose. In these patients, no evidence of vasculitis has been found angiographically, but middle cerebral artery branch occlusion has been demonstrated. (See also cerebrovascular problems due to amphetamines.)

Other rare complications, probably on a vascular basis, include Parkinson's syndrome and hemiballistic movements. Bilateral deafness, either due to anoxia or toxicity, has been observed.

Blindness may occur when quinine has been added to the heroin. This toxic adulterant can also affect the central nervous system; heart, skeletal, and smooth muscles; gastrointestinal tract; kidneys; blood; and the auditory system. Talc emboli in the retinal arteries can cause a field defect or even blindness.

Acute transverse myelitis seems to occur with injected heroin. Sudden paraplegia (occasionally persistent) and thoracic sensory levels characterize this problem, which may be due to a severe systemic reaction to the heroin, quinine, or other adulterants, transient ischemia, hypersensitivity reaction, or a direct toxic effect of the drug.

Peripheral nerve lesions, including brachial and lumbosacral plexitis, atraumatic and traumatic mononeuropathy, and acute and subacute polyneuropathy, may result from direct injection into a nerve or from toxic and allergic reactions. These nerve lesions may also be the sequelae of chronic infection. Atraumatic mononeuropathy, the most frequent neuropathic complication, is characterized by painless weakness beginning 2 to 3 hours after intravenous injection, at a site distal to the injection, and is usually caused by compression of the nerve or its blood supply.

Acute rhabdomyolysis is the most striking type of muscular involvement in heroin abusers. Its onset may occur within a few hours of the intravenous injection of the drug, and it is characterized by skeletal muscle pain and tenderness, swelling, and weakness. Myoglobinemia and myoglobinuria are detected, and acute renal failure may occur.

Chronic fibrosing myopathies are rather common among long-term needle users, probably because of chronic myositis due to brawny edema or a toxic effect of direct intramuscular injection. Unilateral myopathies may be observed in heroin unconsciousness.

Infectious and Postinfectious Neurological Complications

Septic states, with or without endocarditis, can lead to bacterial meningitis and CNS abscesses. In addition, subcutaneous infections may cause peripheral nerve or muscle damage. After fulminating viral hepatitis, there may be a rapid onset of hepatic coma, seizure, decerebrate rigidity, and death 2 to 8 days after onset. The neurological aspects of tetanus are well known.

Neurological Complications of Non-opiate Drugs

Seizures are frequently seen in drug abusers. These can result from overdoses of amphetamines, hallucinogens (LSD), cocaine, and phencyclidine, as well as from opiates. Withdrawal from depressants, including alcohol, can also lead to seizures. The onset of the withdrawal seizures usually occurs 24 to 48 hours after the drug has been stopped, but with longer acting depressants such as diazepam, they can occur 5 to 7 days after withdrawal.

Differentiating between drug-induced seizures and naturally occurring seizures is extremely important both from the standpoint of not missing a treatable neurological disease and not overtreating a drug-induced seizure. Maintenance with Dilantin and/or phenobarbital is not indicated in drug-induced seizures. If, by history, seizures seem related to drug abuse, a trial without antiseizure medication may be useful after the drug abuse has been resolved. Therefore, the following questions are useful diagnostic considerations:

1. What was the temporal relationship between drug use and seizure activity—did the seizure follow the administration of a drug?
2.* Was the use of sedative-hypnotic drugs sufficient to suggest a withdrawal seizure? (See Table 5-1.)
3. Did seizures occur at any time when the patient had been drug-free for several months?

Table 5-1
PHYSICAL DEPENDENCE-PRODUCING DOSAGES OF COMMON SEDATIVE-HYPNOTICS

Drug	Physical dependence-producing dosage (mg daily)	Days needed to produce dependency	Reference	Comments
Secobarbital Pentobarbital	800 or more	35 to 37	Wikler (1968)	Convulsions 2nd to 3rd day of withdrawal
Diazepam	30 or more	42[a]	Pevnick, Jasinski, and Heartzen (1978)	Convulsions 5th to 8th day of withdrawal
Chlordiazepoxide	300 or more	60 to 180	Hollister, Motzenbecker, and Degan (1961)	Convulsions 5th to 8th day of withdrawal
Meprobamate	2400 or more	40[b] to 270[a]	Essig (1964)	Convulsions 2nd to 3rd day of withdrawal

[a]See Smith and Wesson (1974).
[b]See Haizlip and Ewing (1958).

4. Does the EEG show spiking during a period in which the patient has been drug-free for several months? (The EEG is of limited diagnostic value within two weeks after seizure activity or during drug withdrawal or drug intoxication.)

Chronic, intensive alcohol use causes a mixed polyneuropathy sometimes associated with the Wernicke-Korsakoff syndrome. Sniffing gasoline containing lead has resulted in a motor neuropathy or an encephalopathy. Certain solvents such as methylethyl ketone and hexane produce ascending motor polyneuropathy.

A number of cerebral complications of excessive drinking or the associated malnutrition are known: Marchiafava-Bignami disease, the Wernicke-Korsakoff syndrome, pellagra, cerebellar degeneration, and hepatic encephalopathy.

Nystagmus is seen following the use of several different drugs. Nearly all of the depressant drugs cause nystagmus in horizontal gaze, and chronic users may have vertical nystagmus. Phencyclidine also causes horizontal and vertical nystagmus.

Chronic amphetamine use is often characterized by stereotyped behavior. This is manifested by repeatedly performing a task such as picking at the skin. This type of behavior usually disappears after the drug is withdrawn. On withdrawal from prolonged amphetamine use, severe psychomotor retardation and depression may occur and can last for several weeks. This is felt to be secondary to dopamine and norepinephrine depletion. A similar picture (the coke blues) is observed after cocaine discontinuance.

A summary of the physical dependence-producing dosages of common sedative-hypnotic drugs appears in Table 5-1.

Acute intoxication with depressant drugs leads to ataxia as a prominent clinical sign. After prolonged use in some individuals, this ataxia does not clear and may be due to some impairment of cerebellar function. This is most marked in chronic alcohol use where cerebellar atrophy has been described. Cerebral atrophy has been reported as a sequela of almost all forms of drug abuse. However, it has not been sufficiently studied in most drugs to say precisely which drugs may cause atrophy. Chronic use of some solvents has been shown to cause cerebral atrophy in animals, although few cases have been documented in humans. Chronic inhalation of gasoline containing lead has caused lead encephalopathy in the users.

HEMATOPOIETIC COMPLICATIONS

Complications of drug abuse involving the hematopoietic system are seen primarily in those who inject drugs. But drugs taken orally or by inhalation can cause problems with the blood and blood-forming cells. The abuse of drugs containing salicylates—e.g., Darvon compound, Empirin II, etc.—can decrease the number of platelets and lead to bleeding problems. It is important to remember that even though salicylates are not normally considered drugs of abuse, they are often taken in large quantities in over-the-counter medications and in combination with other drugs that have abuse potential.

Abuse of solvents, especially high-dose chronic use, has been associated with bone marrow depression and, in some cases, with aplastic anemia.

Alcohol causes decreased granulocyte adherence, macrocytosis, thrombocytopenia, and decreased levels of reticulocytes and granulocytes in the circulation. This is related to effects on the bone marrow that cause vacuolation of bone marrow pronormoblasts and, in high doses, vacuolation of promyelocytes.

Megaloblastic anemia with leucopenia and thrombocytopenia is a frequent occurrence in alcoholics whose folic acid intake is low. Iron deposits noted in the red blood cell are related to pyriodoxine deficiency.

Bacteremia is the most common of the hematopoietic complications of drug abuse. Caused by repeated unsterile intravenous injections, it is closely associated with the high incidence of infection in other organs. These bacteremias are usually due to normal skin flora, but unusual organisms such as Serratia marcescens can also be found. Associated with the bacteremias is a high incidence of lymphatic lesions. The lymphadenopathy is usually found in nodes located proximally to the injection sites, but also is found in other areas. In cases where lymphadenopathy is found in areas not directly draining injection sites, biopsies should be performed to rule out malignancies.

Upon entering drug treatment programs, most intravenous users are found to have elevations in their immunoglobulins. These are frequently nonspecific but may lead to false positives on many of the routinely performed serological tests. Once illegal drug use stops, most of the elevated immunoglobulin levels return to normal. The high titers of nonspecific immunoglobulin may interfere with specific antibody formation, resulting in the high incidence of infections seen in intravenous drug users.

Recent reports have implicated marijuana as the cause of decreased immunocompetence in chronic users. The primary defect is reported to be in cell-mediated immunity. Whether these changes cause any significant clinical problems is currently being investigated.

Other findings in intravenous drug users are eosinophilia that returns to normal with cessation of drug abuse, and microangiopathic hemolytic anemia.

Chromosomal aberrations have been reported following the use of numerous classes of drugs; LSD has received the most publicity. The data now available on chromosomal damage are conflicting, and the significance of these findings is as yet undetermined.

Autoimmune deficiency syndrome (AIDS) is diagnosed in intravenous drug abusers, especially those injecting heroin or cocaine.

ENDOCRINE COMPLICATIONS

Numerous drugs can cause alterations in endocrine function. Some of the effects of drugs on the reproductive system have already been mentioned. Although not all drugs have been studied for their effects on various hormones, opiates and alcohol have been found to lower testosterone levels. The mechanisms through which these alterations occur are not fully understood and may be different in each case. The testosterone reductions in opiate and alcohol users have been associated with decreased libido and, in some cases, with impotence. Other alterations in endocrine function in opiate users include high resting insulin levels that result in a delayed and smaller rise in insulin levels in a 50 gm oral glucose tolerance test. Growth hormone has also been found to be elevated. Narcotic users have been reported to have elevated thyroxine levels. Cannabis smoking reduces luteinizing hormone levels in males and females.

Substantial alcohol consumption increases the level of adrenocortical hormone and epinephrine secondary to stress. The reduction of available glucose on both a metabolic and nutritional basis can induce alcoholic hypoglycemia. Decompensated diabetes is a late result of severe liver and pancreatic disease.

RENAL COMPLICATIONS

Intravenous heroin use has been reported to be associated with a nephropathy unrelated to bacterial endocarditis. Clinically, this complication presents as a nephrotic syndrome. On renal biopsy, PAS-positive material is seen; and with specific staining, deposits of immunoglobulins are found. This disorder is considered to be an immunologic disorder with the deposition of immune complexes in the glomeruli.

Acute renal failure due to crush injury or overdose, glomerulonephritis due to septic emboli, or necrotizing angiitis with focal renal lesions caused by parenteral amphetamines and possibly heroin are also encountered.

Hesitancy and in some instances prolonged difficulties in initiating micturition have been reported in abuse of narcotic analgesics, amphetamines, and hallucinogens. The effects of these drugs on the bladder and urethra only occur while the drug is in the system. When the effects of the drugs have worn off, this problem is relieved.

SKELETAL COMPLICATIONS

Along with the increased incidence of infections in other organs, the skeletal system should be investigated for septic arthritides and for osteomyelitis. These infections can occur anywhere in the body, and recent reports show that unusual organisms may be present. Low back pain may be due to an infection of the disk space rather than muscle strain.

Crush injuries and fractures are common. The intoxicated individual is more likely to have an accident, and frequently because of the analgesic action of the drug, will not immediately seek treatment. Injuries can also occur with loss of consciousness, causing the patient to sleep in an awkward position that may cut off circulation to an extremity. Frostbite may result from loss of consciousness in the cold.

Intraarterial infections or fasciolitis can cut off circulation to part of an extremity. This can lead to the development of gangrene distally or spontaneous amputation of fingers or toes.

GASTROINTESTINAL COMPLICATIONS

Opiate drugs cause a tonic contraction of the bowel; the result is chronic constipation. This may continue while the patient is in methadone treatment. During withdrawal, diarrhea and abdominal cramping are common.

The stimulant drugs, including the hallucinogens, are anorexiants. In high doses, they can lead to nausea and vomiting. In chronic high-dose amphetamine and cocaine abusers, this can result in severe malnutrition.

Opiates cause spasms of Oddi's sphincter that could lead to cholecystitis in abusers, but this does not appear to be the case; apparently, tolerance develops to this effect. However, drug abusers with a concomitant abuse of alcohol may develop pancreatitis, which in the early stages may mimic the cramps seen in withdrawal. Differentiation can be made by looking for signs of withdrawal other than abdominal cramps. If these are not present, pancreatitis and other abdominal disorders should be considered.

There appears to be a relationship between the drinking of spirits and cancers of the upper digestive tract, especially when smoking is also involved. The alcohol-related increase in gastric acidity accounts for the acute and chronic gastritis and peptic ulceration.

Carbohydrate, specific amino acid, and thiamine malabsorption add to the malnutrition of the chronic alcoholic. Diarrhea and steatorrhea are the result of chronic pancreatitis.

COMPLICATIONS UNRELATED TO DRUG ABUSE

In managing a disease not directly caused by drug abuse, it must be remembered that chronic illness may be complicated by the abuse of drugs.

Diabetes. Diet and hygiene may be neglected—a serious problem in this metabolic disease. Insulin requirements of the diabetic may be affected by alcohol, solvents, and the central stimulants.

Epilepsy. The sedative effects of anticonvulsant medication may be intensified by depressant drug abuse. Withdrawal seizures may be more likely in epileptics.

Hypertension. Stimulants can alter the requirements for antihypertensive medication, causing loss of blood pressure control.

Abdominal pain. In a narcotic abuser, pain may be attributed to withdrawal when, in fact, it may be due to appendicitis, pancreatitis, perforated ulcer, or some other cause of acute abdominal pain.

MATERNAL AND NEONATAL COMPLICATIONS

Although research on the effects of drug abuse during pregnancy and on the offspring of drug abusers has produced some contradictory findings, we do know that pregnancy in the drug abusing woman carries with it potential health problems for mother and child—both before and after birth. Problems arise from the pharmacologic impact of an abused substance on the woman and fetus, as well as from the diluents and routes of administration associated with the nonmedical use of drugs.

Problems also arise from the lifestyle of women who abuse drugs. Very often that lifestyle involves generally poor diet and hygiene, criminal involvement—especially prostitution with a high incidence of venereal disease—and a general lack of prenatal care. Since women of childbearing age represent the vast majority of drug abusing women in treatment, and since the incidence of birth of addicted neonates is increasing, attention to these complications is an important aspect of the diagnosis and evaluation of drug abuse problems among female patients.

COMPLICATIONS DURING PREGNANCY

Malnutrition and all of the illnesses typically associated with drug abuse present particular complications of the pregnant abuser. In addition, the impact of drugs themselves upon the woman and fetus create other major complications. The heroin addicted woman who is not in treatment often goes through withdrawal—possibly because of a lack of drugs or as a result of an attempt to cure her own habit. Dangers to the fetus are significant in this case, for the fetus may well experience withdrawal in utero and could die as a result.

Just as the placenta does not act as a barrier to most drugs of abuse, neither does it protect the fetus from medically prescribed drugs, including methadone. The administration of any drug during pregnancy should, therefore, be undertaken with caution. The particular implications of methadone treatment and withdrawal during pregnancy have been mentioned earlier in our review of systems.

COMPLICATIONS AT BIRTH AND AFTER BIRTH

A significant problem associated with the offspring of drug abusers is the presence of withdrawal syndrome in the newborns of opiate dependent mothers. The greatest danger is that the syndrome may go unrecognized and untreated—resulting at least in the child's suffering and at worst, his or her death. The diagnostic role of the physician treating a possible drug dependent neonate is a critical one. The signs most likely to appear early on in the neonate are irritability; hypertonicity; high-pitched, shrill cries; and tremors. These do not necessarily confirm the existence of dependence and withdrawal, but they do indicate the need for further observation. Other signs include vomiting, hyperactivity, poor food intake, diarrhea, fever, sustained Moro's reflex, and seizures. Suggestive signs include sneezing, respiratory distress, twitching, blueness of skin, yawning, apnea, coryza, tearing, and excessive sweating.

Low birth weight is a frequent occurrence in children of tobacco, cannabis, and heroin dependent mothers. Prematurity usually occurs in 6% to 7% of births; but in heroin addicted mothers about one-third of the babies are premature, with some researchers believing that the rate may be as high as 50%. The low birth weight is of great importance since there is a high correlation between low birth weight and infant mortality.

While the existence of acute symptomatology may last a fairly short period of time, at least one study suggests that infants withdrawn from heroin may experience some disturbances for up to 6 months. Appearance of such signs—particularly in the methadone dependent neonate—may not appear for several weeks after birth. This creates a particularly difficult diagnostic problem, because by the time signs of withdrawal appear, the child may have left the hospital. Care should be taken to attempt to monitor the progress of any infants who are potentially dependent, even though signs do not appear immediately after birth.

The physician should be aware that drugs used frequently to treat withdrawal in the neonate, i.e., phenobarbital and paregoric, can also cause dependence. Therefore, treatment with these drugs should not be prolonged. Otherwise, once the immediate problem has been controlled, the infant might have to be detoxified from the drugs used to treat the original withdrawal.

A neonatal withdrawal syndrome may occur with depressants, including ethanol. Some research has indicated that fetuses of alcoholic mothers may show prenatal and postnatal growth deficits, developmental delay and retardation, microcephaly, short palpebral fissures, maxillary hypoplasias, altered palmar creases, cardiac anomalies, poor motor function, and anomalous external genitalia. Low birth weight and small size are more common findings. Of less frequent occurrence are epicanthi, micrognathia, cleft palate, flattened philtrum, hip dislocation, elbow limitation, phalangeal anomalies, capillary hemangiomas, and rarely, excessory nipple and asymmetrical ptosis. Babies may resemble those with the Cornelia de Lang syndrome. The father's contribution to these signs is under study. This collection of signs or partial expressions of them is known as the fetal alcohol syndrome (FAS). A similar picture, although less frequent, has been described for neonates whose mothers deny alcohol intake during pregnancy, but admit to moderate or heavy marijuana smoking.

One accompanying problem of maternal drug abuse is the apparent frequency with which infants and children die suddenly at home. Again, the research is so sketchy that the exact relationship between death among children and parental drug abuse is unclear. However, in his or her role as diagnostician, the physician should alert both male and female patients that threats to offspring may exist in the home and he or she should assist the parents in identifying such threats. Any such indications warrant the inclusion of family counseling or other social services as a part of the patient's treatment plan. The burden is on the physician to emphasize the importance of postnatal visits.

REFERENCES

Essig, C. F. Addiction to nonbarbiturate sedative and tranquilizing drugs. *Clinical Pharmacology and Therapeutics,* 1964, *5,* 334-343.

Haizlip, T. M., & Ewing, J. A. Meprobamate habituation: A controlled clinical trial. *New England Journal of Medicine,* 1958, *258,* 1181-1186.

Hollister, L. E., Motzenbecker, F. P., & Degan, R. O. Withdrawal reactions from chlordiazepoxide ("Librium"). *Psychopharmacologia,* 1961, *2,* 63-68.

Pevnick, J. S., Jasinski, D. R., & Heartzen, C. A. Abrupt withdrawal from therapeutically administered diazepam: Report of a case. *Archives of General Psychiatry,* 1978, *35,* 995-998.

Smith, D. E., & Wesson, D. R. *Diagnosis and treatment of adverse reactions to sedative-hypnotics* (Department of Health, Education and Welfare Publication No. (ADM) 75-144). Washington, D.C.: U.S. Government Printing Office, 1974.

Wikler, A. Diagnosis and treatment of drug dependence of the barbiturate type. *American Journal of Psychiatry,* 1968, *125,* 758.

6
Helpful Diagnostic Tests

Determining the presence or absence of physical dependence on a given drug is important, but it is not the *most* important factor in assessing a patient at the pretreatment stage. If the patient is in withdrawal when he or she applies for treatment, an experienced clinician can usually identify objective signs that can be rated. For narcotics, the Himmelsbach Rating Scale, which rates the severity of withdrawal in a narcotic dependent individual, has been useful. Unfortunately, objective signs are not always present. This is particularly true if, before coming to the clinic, an abuser has injected narcotics in a quantity great enough to relieve withdrawal symptoms but not cause intoxication.

TESTING WITH NALOXONE

A test using the short-acting narcotic antagonist naloxone eliminates some of the problems of the nalorphine test (nalorphine produces its own narcotic symptoms, confusing the test results; it also produces respiratory depression). Even so, many variables still must be controlled. *This test should not be used in pregnant drug dependent individuals, since it may induce abortion.*

Investigations are currently underway to develop quantitative information about naloxone to make this test more useful. It should be remembered that the severity of physical dependence does *not* necessarily correlate with the severity of psychological dependence. Thus, the patient can be psychologically dependent and not physically dependent and vice versa. Also, a positive opiate urine test says nothing about physical dependence; it only indicates recent drug use.

No simple test like the naloxone test is available to determine if physical dependence exists for drugs other than opiates. One method that is used is to withhold giving any drug to the patient and observe, looking for clinical signs of withdrawal. Another method is to administer a short-acting drug of the same class of drugs to which physical dependence is believed to exist. Since tolerance develops to most drugs to which physical dependence develops, the patient will be able to take a standard dose or more of the drug without showing any clinical signs of intoxication. For example, in depressant dependence, a short-acting barbiturate such as pentobarbital can be administered every hour until signs of intoxication are seen. The more drug needed to produce intoxication, the greater the degree of dependence. If intoxication occurs on the first dose, the patient is not dependent on depressants.

The naloxone test is a safe, rapid, effective, and inexpensive method of diagnosing the physical dependence of a patient on heroin, morphine, and methadone. The test can be accomplished with a minimum of personnel. Unlike urinalysis, it distinguishes between physical dependence and simple use by the patient, and it takes only 10 to 35 minutes. *The test is not necessary in patients displaying signs of withdrawal.*

THE PROCEDURE

After a complete history has been taken and a physical examination performed, the physician records:

1. Pulse
2. Oral temperature
3. The presence of piloerection on the thorax
4. Lacrimation
5. Rhinorrhea
6. Blood pressure
7. Pupil size (measured to 0.2 mm)
8. Sweating
9. Yawning
10. Subjective complaints

A dose of 0.16 mg (0.4 ml) of naloxone hydrochloride is then given intramuscularly in the triceps. After 20 to 30 minutes, the previous observations are repeated and recorded. If no piloerection is present, a second dose of 0.25 mg (0.6 ml) of naloxone hydrochloride is given, this time intravenously. In 2 minutes, the above observations are again repeated and recorded.

A positive naloxone test indicates the presence of physical dependence on opiates and is characterized by the following clinical signs:

1. Increase in pulse rate
2. A fall in temperature
3. Increase in pupil size
4. Sweating
5. Lacrimation
6. Rhinorrhea
7. Elevation of blood pressure
8. Piloerection on the chest
9. Yawning

Attempts have been made to correlate results of the naloxone test with extent of dependence. This is difficult because the time since the last dose of narcotics is an uncontrollable variable, and the severity of dependence cannot be noted by a simple extrapolation from the naloxone response.

In performing the test, it is important to differentiate between the clinical signs described and subjective complaints. This comes with experience. Some clinicians have administered a placebo in order to assist in this differentiation. A consent form should be signed by the patient prior to the administration of naloxone or a placebo.

At present, it is suggested that the naloxone test be used only to exclude the presence of physical dependence in applicants for methadone therapy who may have needle tracks and a positive urine but no signs of withdrawal.

TESTS FOR ALCOHOL DEPENDENCE

For use with the patient suspected of dysfunctional drinking, self-assessment and alcoholism rating scales are available. The most widely used of these is the Michigan Alcoholism Screening Test (MAST) (Selzer, 1971). A shorter version, the SMAST, is also helpful (Selzer, Vinokur, & van Rooijen, 1975).

No reliable biological marker for diagnosing alcoholism exists at this time. The most sensitive test is the GGT (also called the GGTP), the gamma glutamyltranspeptidase test, a liver enzyme. It is not specific for alcoholic liver damage but is quite useful. Other liver enzyme studies, like the SGOT, are also helpful. Triglyceride levels provide substantiating information. In addition, uric acid levels are elevated in some people during and shortly after drinking bouts. Macrocytosis, as measured by the mean corpuscular volume, is sometimes present in heavy users of alcohol.

The blood alcohol level (BAL) is only indicative of very recent drinking. However, a person appearing for a general medical examination with a BAL of more than 100 mg/dl, or someone with a BAL of 150 mg/dl without signs of intoxication (evidence of tolerance), or someone with a BAL of 300 mg/dl at any time, is presumed to be an alcoholic (Morse & Hurt, 1979).

LABORATORY TESTS

Each patient being evaluated for possible treatment in a drug abuse program should have a battery of diagnostic tests performed; these aid in the diagnosis of drug abuse as well as uncover possible medical complications of that abuse. Each patient should have his or her urine checked for drugs to determine which drugs have been used recently. A urinalysis should be performed to uncover a possible nephropathy. Blood studies should include a CBC, SMA12 serology, and Australia antigen. (A positive serology should be further evaluated with a Fluorescent Treponema Antibody [FTA] test, since false positives are common.) A chest X-ray should be taken if this has not been done in the past 6 months. An EKG should be performed on patients over 35, or if there is a history of heart disease in younger patients. If there is a history of seizures, whether associated with withdrawal or not, an EEG should be performed. Additional laboratory tests may be ordered depending on the findings of the history and examinations. In female patients, a Pap smear should be taken during vaginal examination if none has been taken in the past 6 months. Culture for gonorrhea should be collected routinely. Pregnancy tests should be performed in patients who have missed their last menstrual periods or who have irregular menstrual cycles.

Urine testing for drugs is the most common method used in drug abuse centers. Alcohol is routinely checked with breath analyzing devices that automatically convert breath alcohol to blood alcohol concentrations.

It has become commonplace to employ immunoassays such as the EMIT system (Syva) or the RAI system (Roche Diagnostics) on urine samples obtained under observation. These are excellent screening devices for THC, the common opiates, sedatives, stimulants, and PCP. They should be confirmed by gas chromatography or by more sophisticated chromatographic procedures if legal or disciplinary consequences are involved. It should be emphasized that a simple marijuana cigarette may produce a positive for THC 72 hours after smoking, therefore it is not diagnostic of acute intoxication.

A recent development has been the combined use of the SMA12, the SMA6, and the complete blood count as a method for establishing a diagnosis of early alcoholism. These tests are routinely requested and do not add to patient costs. Utilizing this battery of twenty-five tests and applying a quadratic discriminant analysis to the data, Ryback et al. were able to predict 94% of alcoholics in treatment programs and 100% of nonalcoholics correctly. Sixteen of the twenty-three alleged nonalcoholics who drank more than three drinks a day were also found to give positive results. The test was not accurate for those over 65 years of age. As the statistical software for the test becomes available, it may become a valuable screening device in physicians' offices and hospital admission services.

CONSIDERATIONS FOR EVALUATION

After compiling the information from the physical examination, patient interview, and laboratory tests, the physician can design a treatment plan based on the information gathered—for example, the levels of physiological and psychological dependence, the drugs that the patient is abusing, and the accompanying medical problems that may require treatment.

Once the information has been gathered there are several important questions that the physician should ask himself or herself:

1. Does the information gathered from the patient indicate the use of a particular treatment regimen because of drug use, age, sex, treatment history, or family background?

2. Does the information indicate that the patient has problems beyond the scope of the available drug treatment programs—for example, treatment setting, or serious medical problems that could not be handled in the treatment program's setting?
3. Are there factors that predate the drug abuse behavior that cannot be addressed by attacking the patient's drug abuse problems themselves—for example, sexual or social dysfunction that arose long before the drug abuse?

REFERENCES

Morse, R. M., & Hurt, R. D. Screening for alcoholism. *Journal of the American Medical Association,* 1979, *242,* 2688-2690.

Ryback, R. S., Edkhardt, M. J., & Pautier, C. P. *Biochemical and hematological correlates of alcoholism.* R.C.C.P.P., 1982.

Selzer, M. L. The Michigan Alcoholism Screening Test: The quest for a new diagnostic instrument. *American Journal of Psychiatry,* 1971, *127,* 1653-1658.

Selzer, M. L., Vinokur, A., & van Rooijen, L. A. A self-administered Short Michigan Alcoholism Screening Test (SMAST). *Journal of Studies on Alcohol,* 1975, *36,* 117-126.

7
Diagnosis Posttest

Answers to the Posttest appear on page 77.

PART I. TRUE-FALSE QUESTIONS
DIRECTIONS: For each statement below, place a check mark next to the "T" if the statement is true, or next to the "F" if it is false.

1. Most of the cases of tetanus in the United States are found in drug abusers.

   T _____   F _____

2. Impulse control is not a prognostic indicator of success in substance abuse intervention treatment.

   T _____   F _____

3. When acute transverse myelitis is found among the drug-using population, it usually occurs with amphetamine users.

   T _____   F _____

4. Contact dermatitis may result from continued use of topical antiseptics prior to injection.

   T _____   F _____

5. The physician can safely assume that severe mood swings among known drug abusers are drug induced.

   T _____   F _____

6. The physician who finds lymphadenopathy in an area not directly draining an injection site can reasonably assume that **no** malignancy is present.

   T _____   F _____

7. Diminished testosterone levels among alcoholics are caused by concurrent action upon the liver and the testes.

   T _____   F _____

8. The presence of a severe psychological disturbance is one important reason for drug abuse treatment failure.

   T _____   F _____

9. Assessment of suicidal potential should have two concerns: (1) immediate risk, and (2) potential under stressful emotions occurring during treatment.

   T _____   F _____

10. The diabetic's insulin requirements are not affected by drugs that are abused.

    T _____   F _____

11. Symptoms present in primary depression and withdrawal from stimulants are similar.

    T _____   F _____

12. Marijuana is reported to increase testosterone levels while concurrently diminishing sperm counts.

    T _____   F _____

13. When a pregnant heroin addicted woman **not** in treatment goes through withdrawal, effects on the fetus are negligible.

    T _____   F _____

14. Because "junk" hepatitis is caused by contaminated materials in the liver, it has a different outcome than other forms of hepatitis.

    T _____   F _____

15. The physician is right in assuming that abdominal pain in a drug abuser is a symptom of withdrawal.

    T _____   F _____

16. Hyperpigmentation may result from carbon deposits associated with needle sterilization.

    T _____   F _____

17. Epileptic drug abusers are no more likely than other drug abusers to be subject to seizures during drug withdrawal.

    T _____   F _____

PART II. MULTIPLE CHOICE QUESTIONS

DIRECTIONS: Each question below has four or five answers. Pick the **one** answer to each question that is **most true** and place a check mark in front of that answer.

18. In the emergency diagnosis of drug overdose, pupillary constriction can be an indicant of—

    _____ A. Ethanol.
    _____ B. Narcotics.
    _____ C. Barbiturates
    _____ D. Phenothiazines.
    _____ E. Cocaine.

19. Are any of the following proof of physical dependence on opiates?

    _____ A. The patient says he or she cannot get along without the drug.
    _____ B. Needle tracks are found.
    _____ C. Morphine or quinine is found in the blood.
    _____ D. None of the above.
    _____ E. All of the above.

20. The prime means of detecting serum hepatitis in drug abusers is—

    _____ A. The Australia antigen.
    _____ B. Histologic examination of the liver.
    _____ C. Yellow coloring of the sclera.
    _____ D. None of the above.

21. Needle track scars—

    ____ A. May be found on the body at any site giving access to veins.
    ____ B. Are invariably found on the thighs.
    ____ C. Are invariably found on the arms.
    ____ D. Are invariably of dark pigmentation.

22. Which of the following is **not** associated with a stimulant overdose.

    ____ A. Hypertension.
    ____ B. Anorexia.
    ____ C. Tremors.
    ____ D. Piloerection.
    ____ E. Paresthesia

23. In drug-produced seizures—

    ____ A. Maintenance with Dilantin is usually indicated.
    ____ B. Maintenance with phenobarbital is usually indicated.
    ____ C. Maintenance with methadone is usually indicated.
    ____ D. All of the above are true.
    ____ E. None of the above is true.

24. Spiking of the EEG is a major diagnostic indicator with reference to idiopathic epilepsy—

    ____ A. At least 1 week after the last seizure activity.
    ____ B. During drug withdrawal.
    ____ C. During drug intoxication.
    ____ D. At least several months after the patient has become drug free.
    ____ E. During a seizure.

25. Seizures most often can be produced by—

    ____ A. Use of even low doses of stimulants.
    ____ B. Withdrawal from sedative-hypnotics.
    ____ C. Withdrawal from psychedelics.
    ____ D. All of the above are true.
    ____ E. None of the above is true.

26. Which of the following is **not** a sign of opiate intoxication?

    ____ A. Nodding.
    ____ B. Hypotension.
    ____ C. Hyperthermia.
    ____ D. Miosis.

27. Which of the following is **not** associated with chronic, intensive alcohol use?

    ____ A. Wernicke-Korsakoff syndrome.
    ____ B. Hepatic encephalopathy.
    ____ C. Cerebellar degeneration.
    ____ D. Megoblastic anemia.
    ____ E. All of the above are associated with chronic alcohol use.

PART III. MATCHING QUESTIONS

A. DIRECTIONS: For each numbered set of symptoms, signs, and diagnostic indicators given below, select the **one** lettered heading that **most** closely applies and place a check mark in front of the corresponding letter.

    A. Withdrawal from stimulants
    B. Intoxication with depressants
    C. Intoxication with PCP
    D. Intoxication with opiates/opioids
    E. Intoxication with stimulants

28. Tactile hallucinations, paranoid ideation, elevated heart rate.

    ____ A ____ B ____ C ____ D ____ E

29. Diplopia, dysmetria, hypotonia.

    ____ A ____ B ____ C ____ D ____ E

30. Muscle spasms (or rigidity), analgesia (pin prick), inability to speak.

    ____ A ____ B ____ C ____ D ____ E

74 / *The Diagnosis and Treatment of Drug and Alcohol Abuse*

31. Psychomotor retardation, depressed mood, hyperphagia.

   ____ A ____ B ____ C ____ D ____ E

32. Restlessness, picking at skin, suspiciousness.

   ____ A ____ B ____ C ____ D ____ E

33. Sleepiness, slow and shallow respiration, hypotension.

   ____ A ____ B ____ C ____ D ____ E

34. Paradoxical excitement, dizziness, ataxia.

   ____ A ____ B ____ C ____ D ____ E

35. Dizziness, nystagmus, slurred speech.

   ____ A ____ B ____ C ____ D ____ E

36. Hyperphagia, fatigue, depressed affect.

   ____ A ____ B ____ C ____ D ____ E

37. Sleepiness, pinpoint pupils, hypothermia.

   ____ A ____ B ____ C ____ D ____ E

38. Deep tendon reflexes increased, muscle rigidity, coma.

   ____ A ____ B ____ C ____ D ____ E

B. For each numbered set of symptoms, signs, and diagnostic indicators given below, select the **one** lettered heading that **most** closely applies and place a check mark in front of the corresponding letter.

   A. Overdose of stimulants
   B. Intoxication with hallucinogens
   C. Withdrawal from opiates/opioids
   D. Withdrawal from depressants

39. Motor seizures, orthostatic hypotension, tremors.

   ____ A ____ B ____ C ____ D

40. Marked chilliness, diarrhea, generalized aches.

_____ A   _____ B   _____ C   _____ D

41. Elevated blood pressure, elevated heart rate, synesthesia.

_____ A   _____ B   _____ C   _____ D

42. Arrhythmia, diarrhea, paranoid psychosis.

_____ A   _____ B   _____ C   _____ D

PART IV. MULTIPLE TRUE AND FALSE

DIRECTIONS: Each of the following items has four choices, one of which may be correct, two of which may be correct, three of which may be correct, or all of which may be correct. Using the following key, place the appropriate letter in front of each of the following numbered items.

- A. Only 1, 2, and 3 are correct
- B. Only 1 and 3 are correct
- C. Only 2 and 4 are correct
- D. Only 4 is correct
- E. All are correct

DIRECTIONS SUMMARIZED				
A	B	C	D	E
1,2,3 only	1,3 only	2,4 only	4 only	All are correct

_____ 43. Thought disorders are often times found in—

(1) Schizophrenia.
(2) Organic brain syndrome.
(3) Toxic reaction.
(4) Simple depression.

____ 44. Nystagmus may be found during—

   (1) Alcohol withdrawal.
   (2) PCP intoxication.
   (3) Depressant intoxication.
   (4) Stimulant withdrawal.

____ 45. Neonate withdrawal syndrome is most often associated with—

   (1) Stimulants.
   (2) Depressants.
   (3) PCP.
   (4) Opiates.

____ 46. An inability to achieve orgasm may occur during—

   (1) PCP intoxication.
   (2) Depressant intoxication.
   (3) Stimulant intoxication.
   (4) Alcohol intoxication.

____ 47. Which of the following is associated with the "fetal alcohol syndrome"?

   (1) Pre- and postnatal deficits.
   (2) Low birth weight.
   (3) Retardation.
   (4) Macroencephaly.

____ 48. For which of the following is a urine screen a useful diagnostic aid?

   (1) Stimulant withdrawal.
   (2) Opiate withdrawal.
   (3) Hypnosedative withdrawal.
   (4) Hallucinogen withdrawal.

____ 49. Which of the following are sequelae of drug abuse?

   (1) Abscess.
   (2) Ulceration.
   (3) Infection.
   (4) Wrist scars.

___ 50. Which of the following signs is associated with phencyclidine (PCP) intoxication?

(1) Drooling.
(2) Tachycardia.
(3) Muscle rigidity.
(4) Increased deep tendon reflexes.

DIAGNOSIS POSTTEST ANSWER KEY

Answer	Answer
1. T	26. C
2. F	27. E
3. F	28. E
4. T	29. B
5. F	30. C
6. F	31. A
7. T	32. E
8. T	33. D
9. T	34. B
10. F	35. B
11. T	36. A
12. F	37. D
13. F	38. C
14. F	39. D
15. F	40. C
16. T	41. B
17. F	42. A
18. B	43. A
19. D	44. A

DIAGNOSIS POSTTEST ANSWER KEY (continued)

Answer	Answer
20. A	45. C
21. A	46. C
22. D	47. A
23. E	48. A
24. D	49. E
25. B	50. E

8
Treatment Pretest

Answers to the Pretest appear on page 90.

PART I. MULTIPLE CHOICE QUESTIONS
DIRECTIONS: Each item below has five responses. Pick the **one** response that best answers or completes the question, and place a check mark in front of that response.

1. After obtaining vital signs of a patient admitted for treatment of a drug abuse emergency, the one most important observation for determining therapy is—

    _____ A. Needle tracks on the skin.
    _____ B. Condition of the pupils.
    _____ C. Breath odor.
    _____ D. Breath sounds in the lung.
    _____ E. Assessment of liver size.

2. When methadone is first administered for "street" opiate detoxification, generally—

    _____ A. A single dosage of 20 mg will suppress withdrawal symptoms.
    _____ B. A single dosage of 30 mg will suppress withdrawal symptoms.
    _____ C. 10-mg dosages, repeated every 25 minutes, should be administered until withdrawal symptoms are suppressed.
    _____ D. 20-mg dosages, repeated every 40 minutes, should be administered until withdrawal symptoms are suppressed.
    _____ E. None of the above.

3. At daily dosages of 30 to 40 mg, the weekly decrement for methadone maintenance patients should be—

   _____ A. 2-3 mg weekly.
   _____ B. 2-3 mg biweekly.
   _____ C. 5 mg biweekly.
   _____ D. 5 mg weekly.
   _____ E. 5 mg monthly.

4. Nervousness, anorexia, hypertension, and tremors are symptomatic of—

   _____ A. Stimulant abuse.
   _____ B. Hallucinogen intoxication.
   _____ C. Opiate intoxication.
   _____ D. Alcohol intoxication.
   _____ E. Both A and B.

5. Treatment for hallucinogen intoxication might include—

   _____ A. Sensory stimulation, diazepam, and phenothiazines.
   _____ B. In-depth psychotherapy and phenothiazines.
   _____ C. Low-level sensory stimulation and diazepam.
   _____ D. Phenothiazines alone.
   _____ E. None of the above.

6. To withdraw a patient who is dependent on heroin and barbiturates, the safest technique appears to be to—

   _____ A. Effect immediate "cold turkey" withdrawal for both.
   _____ B. Gradually withdraw both simultaneously.
   _____ C. Give a stabilizing dose of chlordiazepoxide and gradually decreasing dosages of methadone.
   _____ D. Give a stabilizing dose of methadone and gradually decreasing dosages of chlordiazepoxide.
   _____ E. Do none of the above.

7. In the emergency treatment of narcotic overdose, the antagonist of choice is—

    ____ A. Nalorphine (Nalline).
    ____ B. Levallorphan (Lorfan).
    ____ C. Naloxone (Narcan).
    ____ D. Propoxyphene napsylate (Darvon-N).
    ____ E. Naltrexone.

8. The use of diazepam is not recommended during treatment for infant withdrawal because—

    ____ A. Diazepam increases the chance of bilirubin encephalopathy in jaundiced infants.
    ____ B. Diazepam extends the duration of the withdrawal syndrome.
    ____ C. Diazepam is contraindicated with paregoric and chlorpromazine.
    ____ D. Diazepam has a paradoxical effect in neonates.
    ____ E. None of the above.

9. During substitution therapy, 30 mg phenobarbital is administered—

    ____ A. For every 200 mg of short-acting barbiturates.
    ____ B. For every 100 mg of short-acting barbiturates.
    ____ C. On a 1:1 ratio with short-acting barbiturates.
    ____ D. For every 60 mg of short-acting barbiturates.
    ____ E. Never as a substitute for short-acting barbiturates.

10. The principal service a physician in general practice can offer the opioid dependent patient is—

    ____ A. Prescriptions of maintenance levels of methadone.
    ____ B. Prescriptions for analgesics.
    ____ C. Diagnosis and referral to a treatment facility.
    ____ D. The initiation of a treatment program.
    ____ E. The administration of naloxone to assess if the patient is opioid dependent.

11. A physician discovers that his patient on a general medical ward is enrolled in a methadone maintenance program. Which of the following is the best course of action regarding patient management?

82 / *The Diagnosis and Treatment of Drug and Alcohol Abuse*

____ A. Physician should require that the patient be detoxified "cold turkey."
____ B. Physician should proceed to withdraw patient gradually prior to treatment.
____ C. Physician should determine the methadone dosage from patient and initiate treatment.
____ D. Physician should consult treatment program to learn maintenance dose.
____ E. Patient should be transferred to a drug treatment unit for detoxification.

12. In the control of seizures in a patient with status epilepticus, the emergency treatment physician should—

____ A. Give only supportive treatment, since seizures are self-limiting.
____ B. Administer 10 mg I.V. of diazepam, injected rapidly as a single bolus.
____ C. Administer diphenylhydantoin routinely.
____ D. Realize that sedative effects of diazepam may make it difficult to assess mental function in the postseizure period.
____ E. Refrain from giving medications for long-term seizure control.

13. An acceptable procedure for producing emesis in a patient who has orally ingested a substance of abuse less than 1 hour earlier would be—

____ A. 10 ml dose of Ipecac fluid extract (repeated once in 15-20 minutes if emesis does not occur), followed by 1-2 glasses of water several minutes after the Ipecac, to insure that the stomach is not empty.
____ B. 10-30 ml dose of Syrup of Ipecac (repeated once in 15-30 minutes if emesis does not occur), followed by 1-2 glasses of Coca-Cola or other flavored carbonated beverage to kill the taste of the emetic.
____ C. 10-30 ml dose of Syrup of Ipecac (repeated 15-30 minutes if emesis does not occur) followed imme-

diately by activated charcoal 100 g slurry with 250 cc of water.
___ D. 1-3 glasses of fluid, followed by injection S.C. of 6 mg/kg (adult) apomorphine hydrochloride, followed (if necessary) by injection I.V., I.M., or S.C. of a narcotic antagonist to stop the narcotic effects of apomorphine.
___ E. None of the above.

14. The length of time for withdrawal from diazepam to occur following cessation of intake is—

    ___ A. 1 day.
    ___ B. 2-3 days.
    ___ C. 7-10 days.
    ___ D. 3 weeks.
    ___ E. None of the above.

15. Clonidine, as used in treatment of opiate withdrawal, is usually administered—

    ___ A. Once a day.
    ___ B. Two to three times a day.
    ___ C. Once every 72 hours.
    ___ D. Once a week.
    ___ E. None of the above.

PART II. COMPARISON QUESTIONS

DIRECTIONS: In the space provided in front of each numbered word or phrase below, insert:

A, if the item is associated with (A) only
B, if the item is associated with (B) only
C, if the item is associated with both (A) and (B)
D, if the item is associated with neither (A) nor (B)

Questions 16-20

(A) Methaqualone
(B) Glutethimide
(C) Both
(D) Neither

_____ 16. Dialysis may be helpful.

_____ 17. May produce cyclic coma.

_____ 18. Brain stem function is not depressed.

_____ 19. Treat with I.V. fluids and monitor electrolyte balance.

_____ 20. Treat with analeptic drugs.

Questions 21-24

(A) Analgesics
(B) Phenothiazines
(C) Both
(D) Neither

_____ 21. Drug group rarely abused.

_____ 22. Common treatment for chronic abuse of stimulants.

_____ 23. May be used in barbiturate overdose.

_____ 24. May be useful singly or in tandem in case of acute episode in which volatiles have been inhaled.

PART III. MATCHING QUESTIONS
DIRECTIONS: For each numbered sign or symptom of drug overdose, select the **one** lettered heading that most closely applies and place a check mark in front of the corresponding letter.

Questions 25-28

(A) Meperidine
(B) Pentazocine
(C) Dolophine
(D) Narcan
(E) Nalline

25. Most commonly used to maintain the opiate dependent patient and avoid withdrawal during surgery.

   ____ A   ____ B   ____ C   ____ D   ____ E

26. Analgesic agent contraindicated with opiate dependent patient or those maintained on methadone.

   ____ A   ____ B   ____ C   ____ D   ____ E

27. Drug of choice to determine whether patient is opiate dependent.

   ____ A   ____ B   ____ C   ____ D   ____ E

28. May be used for analgesia with methadone-maintained patient.

   ____ A   ____ B   ____ C   ____ D   ____ E

Questions 29-30

   (A) Barbiturates
   (B) Diazepam
   (C) Steroids
   (D) Clonidine

29. Drug of choice in 10-20 mg P.O. dosage for the control of the hyperventilation of acute anxiety.

   ____ A   ____ B   ____ C   ____ D

30. Phenobarbital is administered in substitution therapy.

   ____ A   ____ B   ____ C   ____ D

PART IV. MULTIPLE TRUE AND FALSE

DIRECTIONS: Each of the following items has four choices, one of which may be correct, two of which may be correct, three of which may be correct, or all of which may be correct. Using the following key, place the appropriate letter in front of each of the following numbered items.

   A. Only 1, 2, and 3 are correct
   B. Only 1 and 3 are correct

C. Only 2 and 4 are correct
D. Only 4 is correct
E. All are correct

DIRECTIONS SUMMARIZED					
A	B	C	D	E
1,2,3 only	1,3 only	2,4 only	4 only	All are correct

_____ 31. Characteristics of uncomplicated opiate overdose generally include—

(1) Shallow coma.
(2) Perianal pallor.
(3) Respiration rates between 4-6 per minute.
(4) Muscle tremors.

_____ 32. Characteristics of volatile substance abuse include—

(1) Mucosal blisters in the mouth.
(2) Cardiac arrhythmia.
(3) Mucosal blisters in the nose.
(4) Mild tremors.

_____ 33. Additional causes of coma in alcoholics include—

(1) Cardiac arrhythmia.
(2) Hypoglycemia.
(3) Meningitis.
(4) Subdural hematoma.

_____ 34. In the case of the hyperventilating drug abusing patient without other associated medical conditions causing the hyperventilation—

(1) Oral administration of diazepam (10-20 mg) may prove helpful.

(2) Larger doses of diazepam may be needed for a patient who is a heavy smoker.
(3) The half-life of the administered diazepam is directly proportionate to the patient's years of age.
(4) Treatment with a major tranquilizer is indicated, or is usually indicated.

_____ 35. The emergency management of the suicidal patient—

(1) Requires special skill, which not every therapist or physician may have.
(2) Is made easy by the availability of antidepressant medications.
(3) Should involve psychiatric consultation if there is any doubt as to the degree of depression.
(4) Is not difficult if the attempt was minor or innocuous.

_____ 36. In cases of tricyclic antidepressant overdose—

(1) Effects of these drugs are often quite prolonged.
(2) Blood levels of these drugs are easily detectable.
(3) Experience suggests that physostigmine salicylate can be life-saving.
(4) Early treatment with stimulant medications is indicated.

_____ 37. Methadone maintenance for pregnant women may be advisable because—

(1) Withdrawal from narcotics may result in fetal death.
(2) Prematurity of the newborn is more common to heroin dependent than methadone maintained mothers.
(3) Patients will otherwise continue to use narcotics as well as a variety of other drugs.
(4) "Street" heroin use is associated with 80% greater perinatal morbidity and mortality than is methadone maintenance.

_____ 38. In the treatment of both abstinent and methadone-supported patients, clinical impressions suggest that—

(1) They can be successfully treated in the same unit on an outpatient basis.
(2) They can be successfully treated in the same unit on a residential basis.
(3) "Mixed" programs help many who would not succeed in a "pure" methadone program or a traditional therapeutic community.
(4) "Mixed" programs are less suitable for young polydrug users.

_____ 39. Preferred practice during withdrawal from stimulants is to—

(1) Substitute methylphenidate (Ritalin) and then gradually decrease the dose of Ritalin over a 2-week period.
(2) Use sedative or major tranquilizers, as indicated.
(3) Use tricyclic antidepressant drugs at regular intervals.
(4) Refer patient for long-term care.

_____ 40. During a medical crisis involving a patient on methadone maintenance—

(1) Methadone should be discontinued.
(2) Pentazocine (Talwin) should not be used for analgesia.
(3) If narcotics (e.g., Demerol) are indicated, dosages should be kept lower than normal.
(4) If parenteral administration is necessary, 10 mg of methadone two or three times daily (either I.M. or S.C.) will almost always suffice, regardless of previous oral-dose levels.

_____ 41. Diazepam—

(1) Can be readministered every 20 minutes for persistent seizures.
(2) Is useful as a general anesthetic in seizure treatment.
(3) In 10 mg I.V. dosages is the treatment of choice for status epilepticus.

(4) Is a good antiseizure agent with little sedative properties.

_____ 42. An important emergency procedure for the unconscious patient is to—

  (1) Administer naloxone.
  (2) Obtain blood pressure and treat as needed.
  (3) Monitor urinary output.
  (4) Examine patient for coexisting pathology.

_____ 43. Gastric lavage is contraindicated—

  (1) After overdose with tricyclic compounds.
  (2) Anytime beyond 1 hour after ingestion of strong corrosive agents.
  (3) Anytime within 3 hours after drug ingestion.
  (4) Anytime strychnine or petroleum distillates have been ingested.

_____ 44. Isotonic or one-half isotonic physiological saline solution is recommended for gastric lavage because—

  (1) Electrolyte-free water is capable of initiating, without warning, tonic and clonic seizures with coma (cardinal symptoms of water intoxication).
  (2) Ordinary tap water is unsafe, due to its lack of sterility.
  (3) It is safer for patients (particularly children) who have a limited tolerance for electrolyte depletion.
  (4) There is less danger of aspiration.

PART V. TRUE-FALSE QUESTIONS

DIRECTIONS: For each statement below, place a check mark next to the "T" if the statement is true, or next to the "F" if it is false.

45. Physicians are permitted to provide maintenance levels of any opioid drug to opioid dependent patients in a hospital.

    T _____   F _____

46. Current FDA regulations require that for opiate dependent persons who have been dependent for less than 2 years, detoxification must be completed within 45 days.

    T _____   F _____

47. The most common problem seen in patients on methadone maintenance is the abuse of alcohol.

    T _____   F _____

48. Naltrexone is addicting.

    T _____   F _____

49. Punishment as used in traditional therapeutic communities is an effective method of controlling acting-out behavior in adolescents.

    T _____   F _____

50. The most serious problem in the therapeutic community approach is a high recidivism rate.

    T _____   F _____

TREATMENT PRETEST ANSWER KEY

Answer	Answer
1. B	26. B
2. A	27. D
3. D	28. A
4. E	29. B
5. C	30. A
6. E	31. B
7. C	32. A

TREATMENT PRETEST ANSWER KEY (continued)

Answer		Answer	
8.	A	33.	E
9.	B	34.	A
10.	C	35.	B
11.	D	36.	B
12.	B	37.	A
13.	E	38.	A
14.	C	39.	C
15.	B	40.	C
16.	C	41.	B
17.	B	42.	E
18.	D	43.	C
19.	C	44.	B
20.	D	45.	F
21.	B	46.	F
22.	D	47.	T
23.	D	48.	F
24.	D	49.	F
25.	C	50.	F

9
Responding to Common Emergencies

GENERAL MANAGEMENT OF CRISIS

Crisis intervention is by definition short term; it involves alleviating the distress and confusion of a specific event or circumstance. The conscious patient with drug- or alcohol-related emergency problems is often experiencing severe emotional stress. In some cases, medical or biological solutions will exacerbate rather than alleviate the crisis. In such instances, the most important crisis intervention tools are the verbal and nonverbal communication skills of the attending physician.

The goal of crisis intervention is to establish and maintain rapport, create trust, and build a short-term working relationship that will lower anxiety, produce a clearer understanding of the problem at hand, and identify the resources necessary to cope with it.

Psychotherapy, psychoanalysis, and in-depth counseling are not appropriate forms of crisis intervention, although they may be indicated once the resolution of the immediate pain or reaction has occurred. In fact, using the techniques or approaches of long-term, problem solving methods may reduce the effectiveness of the intervention and compound the problem.

GUIDELINES TO CRISIS MANAGEMENT

The following guidelines may be helpful in reducing emotional overreaction by helping the patient make sense out of what is happening to him or her:

1. Provide a reality base.
    a. Identify yourself and your position.

b. Use the patient's name.
   c. Anticipate the concerns of the patient, family, and friends.
   d. Based on the patient's response, introduce as much familiarity as possible, e.g., persons, objects, newspapers, TV programs.
   e. Be calm and self-assured.
2. Provide appropriate nonverbal support.
   a. Maintain eye contact.
   b. Maintain a relaxed body posture.
   c. Touch the patient, if it seems appropriate.
3. Encourage communication.
   a. Communicate directly with the patient, not through others.
   b. Ask clear, simple questions.
   c. Ask questions one at a time.
   d. Try to use open-ended questions.
   e. Tolerate repetition.
4. Foster confidence.
   a. Be nonjudgmental.
   b. Listen carefully.
   c. Respond to feelings.
   d. Identify and reinforce progress.

BEHAVIORAL EMERGENCIES

All drug abuse patients presenting themselves with psychiatric difficulties in the emergency room will demonstrate an acute disturbance in their ability to think, feel, and function. These psychiatric symptoms are present regardless of whether or not they have any kind of underlying medical or psychiatric difficulty.

The psychiatric emergencies of drug abusing patients may be divided broadly between those of the acutely intoxicated state and the more chronic medical, psychological, and social problems of drug abuse. The problems related to acute intoxication should be handled in a clear and systematic fashion because they may be potentially life threatening.

Various psychiatric problems—mental disorders secondary to drug effects, primary mental disorders, suicidal behavior, violent behavior—are common in emergency room settings. However, patients using drugs are less likely to be schizophrenic than under the influence of hallucinogenic drugs, central stimulants, or other medications. They may present with acute psychiatric decompensation, paranoid disorders, or other symptoms. In emergency situations, it may be hard to distinguish among chronic or acute mental problems and those that are drug-related. Furthermore, in an emergency room setting, it is nearly impossible to say with certainty whether the patient has a mental disorder secondary to drug effects or a primary mental disorder.

Patients with mental disorders secondary to drug effects usually demonstrate altered levels of consciousness, fluctuating mental status examinations, and altered vital signs. In addition, there may be disturbances in memory and the ability to concentrate. Patients with primary mental disorders are more rarely disoriented as to time, place, and person than drug abusing patients; have auditory rather than visual hallucinations; and have a slow onset and a relatively constant degree of impairment. From a practical point of view, it may be impossible in the emergency room setting to adequately test for orientation because of the patient's high level of anxiety.

The mental status examination should include tests of orientation, memory (both recent and remote), a description of appearance, level of consciousness, affect, degree of logic, thought content, and some assessment of judgment and insight.

Almost all acutely psychotic patients with alcohol odor or suspected of being under the influence of drugs should be handled in a supportive medical setting until it can be ascertained whether the individual has a primary thought disorder. Providing familiar people and objects may help reduce the patient's anxiety.

A supportive, calm environment for the patient should be provided and serial observations of mental status should be made. If there is no apparent impending medical crisis, the patient should be removed from the crisis environment, careful explanation of the surroundings should be attempted, health personnel should be confident but not overly solicitous, relatives should be contacted, and medical records should be obtained promptly. The patient should be assured that the problem is only temporary, and that he or she will be better shortly. The goal is to make an ongoing reassessment of the patient's mental status and to provide the patient with a controlled, calm, and reassuring environment.

There is a tendency to overmedicate these patients with tranquilizing drugs. In the emergency setting, if it can be done, the best therapy is no pharmacotherapy. If, however, sedative medications must be administered, then oral benzodiazepines (diazepam, 10-30 mg) are preferred initially. Diazepam should not be administered to anyone having a problem with control of impulses. With diazepam, as with alcohol, there is a tendency to lower inhibition; this may make the problem of control more difficult. These drugs have a wide therapeutic margin of safety and will allow for a continued mental status examination for purposes of arriving at a more accurate diagnosis.

If it is clear with psychiatric consultation that a thought disorder is present, then phenothiazine medications, such as chlorpromazine (Thorazine), may be administered four times a day in a dose of 25-50 mg, preferably by mouth. *Chlorpromazine should never be administered intravenously, because of its hypotensive qualities.* Sometimes, however, intramuscular chlorpromazine is needed. If pain or irritation is a problem, dilute with 2% procaine. With initial therapy, there may be atropinic-like side effects, hypotension, or dystonic reactions. Haloperidol (Haldol), another antipsychotic drug with fewer side effects than chlorpromazine, has been found useful in controlling acute psychotic behavior. It can be given in doses of 1-5 mg every 2 hours until a calming effect is achieved.

MANAGEMENT OF THE VIOLENT PATIENT

In management of the violent patient, there are two basic principles that should be practiced. First, do not approach a potentially violent patient alone. Do so only with a sufficient number of people to control an outbreak of violence. Treatment personnel should not create a situation in which they may be injured.

It is important to protect the potentially violent patient as well as the potential victim. Second, avoid aggressive actions unless there is the immediate possibility of serious injury. In all other circumstances, only defensive techniques, e.g., holding the arms or legs, or rolling in a blanket, should be permitted.

If the attending physician is assaulted, it is possible that he or she ignored the many signals of impending loss of control presented by the patient. These include high degrees of agitation, sweating, and excessive talking while struggling with violent impulses, etc. Personnel should be taught to control their own anxiety, to be alert to such signals, and to take evasive action (leaving the room or calling in other people) before the patient's impulses are translated into action. There is nothing wrong with running from an emergency room occupied by a physically threatening patient, armed or unarmed.

If a patient is armed, the police must be called. If there are not enough personnel available to ensure control of an unarmed but violent patient, the police should be called. Once they have neutralized the threat, diagnostic and therapeutic activities can be resumed.

SUICIDE

Drug abusing patients walk a narrow line between mortgaging today's mood effects for tomorrow's medical complications. Failure may precipitate a suicide attempt, but other reasons for suicidal behavior also exist. The management of the suicidal patient requires special skill. Not all therapists or physicians are capable of dealing with the suicidal or depressed patient.

The person who makes a suicide attempt, even though that attempt appears to be minor and innocuous, may be calling for help. The attempt should be taken very seriously; it has great importance to the individual. Discuss the patient's emotional state. Try to find if there is evidence of previous depression or suicidal intent. Seek information about whether the individual made a serious plan for the attempted suicide.

The patient must be protected while in the environment of the treatment room or emergency room setting. Needles, sharp instruments, drugs, etc. should not be in the immediate proximity of the patient. Also, he or she should be observed at all times.

If there is any doubt as to the degree of the depression in the suicidal intent, psychiatric consultation should be obtained. Note, also, that the medications that are useful in treating severe depression take several days to weeks to be effective, and that side effects appear before therapeutic benefits. Patients must, therefore, be placed in a supportive and supervised environment while awaiting a full therapeutic response.

Finally, there are a number of factors that, when present, make the possibility of suicide more or less likely for a patient. These factors are outlined in considerable detail in Griffin (1976).

OBSERVATION AND DIAGNOSIS

A patient's medical history is a major feature of the diagnostic process. The drug abusing patient's history, however, can be unreliable, especially in situations presumably caused by drug abuse. He or she may not want to volunteer appropriate information. Moreover, the drug abuser may be unable to give accurate information regarding the type and dose of the drug, its purity, or the degree of tolerance he or she possesses. Thus, it is essential for the physician to base medical decisions primarily on physical diagnostic criteria and laboratory findings and secondarily on history.

The most important information to be gathered from the emergency patient concerns the level of consciousness and vital signs. The attending physician should describe the severity of the intoxication by observing:

1. Whether the patient is awake and will answer questions.
2. Whether the patient withdraws from painful stimuli.
3. Whether deep tendon reflexes are present.
4. Whether respiration is intact.
5. The circulatory system as it relates to blood pressure, pulse, and cyanosis.

Typically, most patients will fall into one of three categories:

1. *Awake, claiming to have ingested a medicine*—Patient may be questioned and not fall asleep when left alone.
2. *Semicomatose*—Patient will respond appropriately to verbal or noxious stimuli but fall asleep when stimulus is removed.
3. *Comatose*—Patient cannot be aroused to consciousness by verbal or noxious stimuli.

Supportive care should be initiated as soon as possible. It is obvious that many of the procedures can and should be carried out simultaneously by various members of the emergency team. In any case, the immediate objective is to assess cardiopulmonary functioning and to stabilize those functions before other diagnostic and therapeutic measures are instituted. If the physician is confronted with a comatose patient who is apneic, with severe hypotension and absent heart sounds, emergency cardiopulmonary resuscitation must be started immediately despite the lack of a complete or partial diagnosis.

Once the patient's vital signs have been obtained, the single most important observation for determining therapy is the condition of the pupils. For practical purposes, narcotics and organophosphates are the only drugs that cause extremely small pupils. An occasional patient with glaucoma may be on therapy that causes small pupils; a pontine angle cerebral infarction may also cause small pupils. But in a practical, everyday setting, pinpoint pupils (reactive to light) in a comatose patient will strongly suggest narcotic overdose.

The rest of the brief physical examination should include: careful observation of the skin for needle marks, detection of breath odor, assessment of liver size, and listening to breath sounds in the lung. Any evidence of trauma should be recorded in detail. If head trauma is suspected, the tympanic membrane of each ear should be examined to assure that there is no blood behind the drum. This entire evaluation should take no more than 1 to 2 minutes.

In addition to the physical examination, blood samples should be obtained for CBC, glucose, BUN (blood urea nitrogen), electrolytes, blood gases, and whatever toxicology screening is available.

Once the brief initial assessment is completed, three basic questions must be answered:

1. What is the best supportive care?
2. Can the absorption rate of any drug taken orally be decreased?
3. Are there any antidotes that might be useful in this condition?

MANAGEMENT OF SHOCK

Shock is diagnosed when there is a lack of perfusion of vital tissues. It is not specifically diagnosed by a low blood pressure, although this is a common accompaniment. Blood pressure is the product of the cardiac output times the total peripheral resistance. Shock may result from fluid losses, which cause a decrease in cardiac output; by vasodilation, which causes a decrease in the total peripheral resistance; or by direct depression of the cardiovascular function itself. To treat shock appropriately, the specific cause of the phenomenon must be detected.

In the usual case, a diagnosis of shock is made upon observation of low blood pressure and metabolic acidosis; the patient is cold and clammy, may be confused, and has a decreased urine volume. Such a state requires intensive medical intervention. If there is a suggestion that shock is due to an acute allergic reaction, then antihistaminic medications and steroids should be administered immediately. Fluid loss may occur by bleeding into the abdomen, vomiting of blood, or the passage of blood through the rectum. If the heart is embarrassed, then a careful cardiovascular monitoring and treatment is indicated to assure increased perfusion. Blood cultures should be taken to ensure that shock is not due to systemic infection.

In most varieties of shock where there is no obvious heart failure, the procedure is to elevate the patient's legs, lower the head, and increase fluid volume as rapidly as possible. Vasopressor agents, such as levarterenol and dopamine, may be useful in selected circumstances, but they must be monitored carefully, usually in an intensive care unit.

HYPERVENTILATION

Hyperventilation is a common emergency situation in drug abusing patients. It can be a manifestation of acute anxiety, but it also may indicate metabolic acidosis, severe pain, drug withdrawal, salicylate poisoning, or septicemia. When an individual is breathing rapidly, the pCO_2 falls, leading to decreased cerebral blood flow; the resulting alkalosis causes decreased oxygen release. Alkalosis may also affect serum calcium levels and lead to tetany. It is usually valuable, therefore, to perform a Trousseau and Chvostek test to determine any decrease in calcium level.

Intravenous abuse often sends toxic products directly to a patient's lung. If intravenous abuse and the resultant complications are suspected, an arterial blood gas determination will indicate whether decreased oxygen accounts for the hyperventilation. If a low oxygen level is found, then a medical explanation must be sought.

When associated medical conditions causing hyperventilation are ruled out, having the individual count his or her respirations and breathe into a paper bag in a quiet environment together with verbal reassurance will usually suffice. If a satisfactory result does not occur, then the oral administration of diazepam (Valium), 10-20 mg, will be helpful. Individuals who are heavy smokers tend to require two to three times that dose to get the same effect. Also, the half-life of the administered drug is directly proportional to the years of age of the individual. Thus, the half-life is 20 hours for a person who is 20 years old, and 90 hours for a 90-year-old patient.

Often it is difficult to provide a quiet, reassuring environment in an emergency room setting. The hyperventilating patient should be removed from the crisis situation as soon as possible. Hyperventilating patients should not be left alone. Medical personnel should listen (in a nonjudgmental way) to the problems of the patient and should respond to the patient's questions regarding his or her condition in a calm, professional manner.

REFERENCES

Griffin, J. B. The psychiatric examination. In H. K. Walker, W. D. Hall, & J. W. Hurst (Eds.), *Clinical methods: The history, physical, and laboratory examinations*. Boston: Butterworths, 1976.

10
A General Approach to the Comatose and Semicomatose Patient

THE COMATOSE PATIENT

"Coma" here refers to a state of unconsciousness from which a patient cannot be aroused. Calling the patient's name, applying pressure to the sternum, pinching the nipple, applying pressure to the supraorbital bones (dangerous, since the fingers may slip, damaging the globe of the eye), and other routine measures should be employed. If the patient can be aroused and returned to consciousness, a medical history should be obtained along with the recording of vital signs and examination of cardiopulmonary function. In the event the patient cannot be aroused, the following measures should be instituted.

RESPIRATORY SUPPORT

If necessary, clear airway. Tape a short, plastic, oropharyngeal airway in the mouth to prevent the tongue from obstructing the airway if the patient is not to be intubated. If the patient's jaw is locked from muscle spasm—an occasional occurrence—use succinylcholine chloride (Anectine, Quelicin, Sucostrin—40 mg is an average adult dose) to help gain proper access for establishing an airway. Use of succinylcholine (it should be used only by those skilled in intubation and avoided in PCP intoxication) carries the risk of regurgitant vomiting, but this risk must be accepted in view of the primacy of establishing an airway. It should be understood that use of this agent is justified only if respiratory activity is compromised to the point of endangering the life of the patient. The patient's feet should be slightly elevated and he or she should be positioned face down to minimize the risk of aspiration from vomiting. The use of respiratory stimulant drugs carries unacceptable risks and is not recommended.

Blood gas physiology has proved to be particularly effective in determining the degree of severity of the patient's condition. It must be stressed that an understanding of the milieu of the potential drug therapy is essential to plan a course of pharmacotherapy properly. Drug abusing patients in extremis tend to have low serum potassiums, low serum magnesiums, and low serum phosphates. These commonly result from respiratory alkalosis and renal tubular acidosis. Severely ill drug abuse patients must have an arterial blood gas measurement.

Practice and experience with endotracheal intubation and the use of an Ambu bag is essential for the physician treating the emergency drug abuse patient. The causes of an elevated pCO_2, indicating respiratory acidosis, and of low pCO_2, indicating respiratory alkalosis, should be determined. The normal pH is between 7.37 and 7.42. The common causes of an increased pH with a positive base excess (indicating metabolic alkalosis) and of a low pH with a low base excess (indicating metabolic acidosis) must be clearly understood.

A useful review of acid base disorders can be found in Kassirer (1974). Of special note is the fact that respiratory failure (elevated pCO_2) is a laboratory diagnosis except in the most severe cases. A low oxygen tension in an apparently well patient is strong evidence for a serious underlying condition that requires medical explanation.

PERFORMANCE OF OTHER EMERGENCY PROCEDURES

Establish an intravenous line and draw blood for a drug screen, glucose, alcohol (and other drugs, as indicated by the history), CBC, Na, K, calcium, BUN, creatinine, and blood gases, if indicated.

After the blood is drawn, administer slowly I.V. 0.4 mg of naloxone (Narcan). (The pediatric dose is 0.01 mg/kg.) Prompt improvement of the respiratory rate following this administration suggests narcotic overdose. If respiratory improvement is not marked, the dose should be repeated one or two times every 2-3 minutes. If an I.V. line is not available, naloxone may be given I.M. or S.C. Administration of 50 grams of I.V. glucose should be considered. Obviously, if the patient suffers from hypoglycemic coma and responds to intravenous glucose, management should proceed with dietary adjustments, regulation of insulin if the patient is diabetic, etc.

Since we are concerned here with the possibilities of drug overdose, it is important to emphasize that failure to see a prompt response to naloxone in respiratory rate and volume implies that factors other than opiates are involved. If initial administration of 0.4-0.8 mg of naloxone does not improve respiratory rate, proceed as follows:

1. Intubate, if respirations are shallow or less than eight per minute.
2. If the patient has pulmonary edema or is hypotensive, insert a central venous pressure (CVP) line via a peripheral vein. If, as is often the case with heroin addicts, peripheral veins are not available for drawing blood or inserting a CVP, the subclavian, internal jugular, femoral, or scalp veins may be utilized. It may be necessary to do a cutdown.
3. Maintain suction as necessary.

If the patient responds to naloxone, he or she should be kept under observation in the hospital for at least 24 hours. Naloxone is a short-acting drug (30-120 minutes), whereas all of the narcotic drugs have a longer duration of action. This is particularly important when the patient has overdosed with one of the longer acting drugs, such as methadone. If *l*-alpha-acetylmethadol (LAAM) becomes widely available, periods of observation lasting from 72-96 hours will be necessary, as effects of this drug can last for days. A patient may lapse into unconsciousness following a clearing of the sensorium in response to naloxone, even if shorter acting narcotics are involved. Therefore, all narcotic overdose patients should be observed in the hospital for at least 24 hours. If methadone is involved, longer periods are advisable. The family should be instructed to check frequently on the patient's condition for 1-2 days following discharge from the hospital. In addition to the emergency administration of naloxone and glucose, thiamine 100 mg I.V. or I.M. should be given if there is any possibility of acute alcoholic encephalopathy.

EVALUATION AND TREATMENT OF THE CARDIOVASCULAR SYSTEM

Obtain blood pressure and treat as needed. In a healthy young patient, substantial elevations of blood pressure can be managed conservatively. In this regard, medical consultation should be sought. If diastolic blood pressure *exceeds* 150-160 and/or systolic blood pressure *exceeds* 240-250, antihypertensive agents such as nitroprusside, phentolamine (Regitine), or diazoxide (Hyperstat) should be considered, particularly if such levels are sustained for periods in excess of 15-30 minutes. If the patient is hypotensive place him or her in the Trendelenburg position.

Management of hypotension will frequently be corrected by fluid administration, e.g., a rapid infusion of one-half normal saline or Ringer's lactate, monitoring the CVP with close clinical assessment to prevent fluid overload. If there is no response to fluid administration, start intravenous vasopressors such as phenylephrine hydrochloride (Vasoxyl) or other adrenergic drugs.

These may be required if the patient shows signs of profound shock, with tachycardia above 110 beats per minute, prolonged capillary filling time, pallor, or diaphoresis.

Moderate hypotension as low as 80 mm Hg does not necessitate vigorous therapy with vasopressors unless urinary output is depressed. Extremely potent agents, such as levarterenol bitartrate (Levophed Bitartrate), should be used for severe shock. The prepared solution (see *PDR*) should be given I.V. drip, 2-3 ml per minute for the initial dose, and then adjusted to maintain low normal blood pressure. Note that vasoconstrictors may significantly depress urinary output.

If the patient has no blood pressure or pulse, begin cardiopulmonary resuscitation immediately. Also monitor the electrocardiogram as soon as possible and treat arrhythmias specifically. This is particularly important in an antidepressant overdose, because death has been reported as a result of associated arrhythmias. (NOTE: Arrhythmias may result from prolonged hypoxia, acidosis, cocaine, amphetamine, atropinic agents, volatiles, antidepressants, phenothiazines, and other drugs.)

OTHER MEASURES

Insert indwelling Foley urinary catheter to monitor urinary output. If urine is obtained, save for drug analysis. An endotracheal tube should be placed and the cuff blown up. A nasogastric tube should be inserted and the gastric contents emptied. The stomach should be lavaged, unless lavage is contraindicated. Activated charcoal, 100 mg as a slurry with 250 cc of water, may be instilled into the stomach after lavage has been completed. It can be administered through the lavage tube and then the tube withdrawn.

FURTHER EVALUATION OF THE PATIENT

Routine emergency procedures demand that, after evaluation of the patient's respiratory and cardiovascular systems, there should be an examination and evaluation of the rest of the patient. Failure to do this in the case of unconscious patients suspected of drug overdose has caused serious problems to the patient, to the person(s) providing treatment, and to the institution involved. Routine emergency procedures demand recognizing that:

1. Unconsciousness may result from something other than drug abuse, although the patient may be an abuser. These circumstances include diabetic ketoacidosis, subdural hematoma, etc.
2. There may be coexisting pathology:
   a. Patient may have a fractured hip from a fall.
   b. Patient may have a head injury.
   c. Patient may have trauma only, without drug abuse causing comatose state.

MANAGEMENT OF CONVULSIONS

For the physician providing emergency treatment to drug abusing patients, epilepsy and drug withdrawal seizures are common problems. In the classic circumstance, an epileptic problem begins in childhood. If convulsions occur in adult life, they may be associated with head trauma or acquired central nervous system disorder. However, sedative-hypnotic drugs and alcohol can cause seizures as a manifestation of their withdrawal phenomena.

The most common type of seizure disorder that is a medical emergency is the grand mal seizure. This is a tonic, clonic spasm that usually lasts from 1-2 minutes. During grand mal convulsions, patients are not awake. After the seizure, the patient is confused and weak.

Focal seizures are uncommon in drug withdrawal seizures. Patients who are undergoing withdrawal from a drug (or drugs) and who are having marked tremulousness and anxiety are rarely actually having a seizure.

Occasionally, drugs themselves cause seizures. Seizures may occur with an overdose of methaqualone (Quaalude), heroin, meperidine, phenothiazines, phencyclidine, or stimulants. Hypoxia also may result from any drug overdose and may cause seizures. In addition, acute withdrawal from alcohol, barbiturates, nonbarbiturate hypnotics, and minor-tranquilizers are a frequent cause of drug-related seizures.

For the patient suffering convulsions, a quick physical examination is essential, and he or she must be protected from aspirating. Ventilation must be maintained. The patient should also be protected from self-injury by being placed on the floor or in a bed with side rails. An intravenous line must be supplied. No restraint of movement should be attempted while the patient is convulsing; tight clothing should be loosened. A blood sugar sample should be taken and intravenous sugar administered. It is also good practice to administer vitamin therapy, especially thiamine, to potentially malnourished drug or alcohol abusing individuals.

With a single seizure, it is not necessary to treat the convulsion per se. Following the seizure, however, the drug withdrawal and/or epilepsy should be treated in the usual way. In status epilepticus (repeated seizures without a lucid interval between seizures), however, intravenous diazepam 10 mg is the treatment of choice. The drug should be administered slowly as cardiac arrest may occur. If seizures persist, the diazepam can be administered every 20 minutes. Diazepam is effective, but it is also a sedative drug. Thus, it may be difficult to assess mental function in the postseizure period. Phenytoin (Dilantin) has little sedative property and also has good antiseizure activity. This drug, however, requires a large loading dose, usually in the range of 600 to 1,000 mg given intravenously in 100 mg bolus injections. Intramuscular administration is not appropriate because of poor and irregular absorption. Because phenytoin is a long-acting medication, it is not routinely given unless the seizures are difficult to control.

Regardless of which drug is used, one must always be alert for cardiopulmonary arrest. If it is certain that the patient has epilepsy and has not been taking medication, institution of long-term seizure control should begin, usually with Dilantin, measuring the blood level of the drug and adjusting dosages accordingly. If status epilepticus occurs and is not responsive to diazepam or phenytoin, then general anesthesia with thiopental (Pentothal) should be administered by an anesthesiologist.

In summary, when treating the emergency drug abusing patient who is having convulsions, the physician's primary goal is to prevent physical injury and to assure a patent airway for the patient. The seizure patient should be kept from doing harm to himself or others; aspiration should be prevented at all costs. A quick physical assessment must be made to establish the possibility of metabolic or thermal imbalances. The physician must be able to prepare an intravenous line quickly. A blood sugar should be drawn and intravenous glucose administered to most seizure patients. The physician should have appropriate medications to treat cardiopulmonary arrest, should it occur.

Clear guidelines for nonphysicians should be established for responding to a diagnosis of status epilepticus and for situations requiring anesthesiology or neurosurgical and neurological consultations. Extra caution should be exercised if there is known hepatic or renal disease.

THE SEMICOMATOSE PATIENT

This discussion concerns the patient who is somnolent (sleepy but can be aroused). As the patient who can be aroused may be developing a comatose state, close monitoring is essential.

The patient should be made to walk without assistance, if possible, to maintain a waking state. While the patient is walking, a history can be obtained and appropriate measures taken.

Patients should be observed for 24 hours in the hospital following recovery of full consciousness. This is necessary because of the long-acting nature of some substances, e.g., methadone and meprobamate (Miltown, Equanil), and because of the idiosyncrasies of some drugs, such as the coma and wakefulness cycle seen in glutethimide (Doriden) overdose. Patients who can be aroused should have a complete workup, including history and physical examination, CBC, urinalysis, and chest film, with blood or urine tested to confirm the drug involved.

MANAGEMENT OF ORALLY INGESTED DRUGS

If a drug like alcohol has been taken by mouth and within 1 hour, or if the drug involved is known to cause delayed gastric emptying (e.g., methadone and tricyclic antidepressants), or if the stomach is enlarged to percussion and/or palpation, emesis or gastric lavage should be considered.

EMESIS

Syrup of Ipecac (not the fluid extract, which is fourteen times more potent and extremely toxic) can be given in doses of 10-30 ml and repeated once in 15-30 minutes if emesis does not occur. The patient should also be given fluid (one to two glasses) several minutes after the Ipecac is swallowed, as emesis may not occur if the stomach is empty. (Never substitute carbonated drinks for water.)

If Ipecac does not induce vomiting, gastric lavage becomes doubly imperative because (a) Ipecac left in the stomach is an irritant; and (b) when absorbed, it is a specific cardiotoxin capable of producing disturbances of conduction, arterial fibrillation, or fatal myocarditis. If more than an hour has elapsed since the patient ingested an antiemetic drug, Ipecac should not be used: use gastric lavage instead.

Never give activated charcoal simultaneously with syrup of Ipecac, as it will absorb the Ipecac and prevent its emetic effect. The charcoal can be given safely and should be given after vomiting has completely subsided. Contraindications to using Ipecac are the same as those for gastric lavage.

A widely accepted method used in many poison control centers starts with injecting apomorphine hydrochloride (6 mg for an adult; 0.06 mg for a child) subcutaneously for prompt emesis. This can be followed, if necessary, by naloxone hydrochloride (Narcan), 0.01 mg/kg intravenously, intramuscularly, or subcutaneously, to stop the narcotic effect of the apomorphine. The use of narcotic antagonists is rarely necessary.

For best results (as with Ipecac), give fluids beforehand (one to three glasses), since emesis does not occur readily if the stomach is empty. Apomorphine has three very distinct advantages:

1. Rapid vomiting (within 3-5 minutes) with emptying of all gastric contents.
2. No obstruction of lavage tubes which may produce delays and incomplete emptying.
3. Reflux of contents (enteric-coated tablets, etc.) from the upper intestinal tract into the stomach.

However, do not use apomorphine if the patient is comatose and/or has a significantly depressed cough reflex, or if the injection apomorphine solution is green (this indicates decomposition and the use of an old, outdated tablet).

GASTRIC LAVAGE

If vomiting cannot be induced or is contraindicated, begin gastric lavage at once. Gastric lavage is clearly indicated any time up to 3 hours after the drug has been taken or even later if the stomach is full, if large amounts of milk or cream have been previously taken, or if the drug is enteric coated. Some drugs are reexcreted in the stomach or slowly absorbed, e.g., tricyclic compounds, phencyclidine, and methyl salicylate. If the patient has taken one of these, gastric lavage (or continuous gastric lavage) is warranted even several hours after ingestion. However, there are situations where gastric lavage is contraindicated.

1. Ingestion of strong corrosive agents, such as alkali (concentrated ammonia, lye, etc.) or mineral acids. Note that with ingestion of strong corrosive agents, lavage can be carried out safely within 1 hour of ingestion. This probably should be done to prevent serious caustic burn of the stomach or esophagus followed by ulceration, constriction, or even stenosis.
2. Ingestion of strychnine (a convulsion may be induced if much time has elapsed).
3. Ingestion of petroleum distillates (kerosene, mineral oil).
4. Presence of coma with depression of the cough reflex (aspiration pneumonia may occur).

Gastric lavage can be carried out safely on comatose patients in a hospital or emergency room setting with an endotracheal tube and inflation cuff.

If the patient is a child, the only equipment needed is a common urethral catheter (8-12 F) and a syringe (20 or 50 ml). Plastic duodenal tubes are preferable, however, because of their durability, flexibility, and ease of passage without lubrication. For adults, a tube with a diameter of about 1 cm (between 1/16 and 1/12 inch), 24 F or greater, is usually satisfactory. The larger the tube that can be passed, the more rapidly the lavage can be completed.

In older children and adults, the nasal route is preferred. However, the oral passage is easier and less traumatic for infants and young children. Mark the distance from the bridge of the nose to the tip of the xiphoid process on the lavage tube with adhesive tape prior to passage. Passage will be easier if the tube is immersed in cold water or a water-miscible jelly (avoid oils). (Dentures and other foreign objects should be removed from the mouth; restraints will be needed for most children.) Double-lumen tubes are preferred to single-lumen tubes by many.

In large centers where anesthesiologists are readily available, the patient can be lightly anesthetized, given succinylcholine chloride, and lavaged after an endotracheal tube with an inflated cuff has been inserted into the trachea. (This method, though ideal, would be impractical in most community treatment centers.) The patient should be placed on his or her left side, with head hanging face down over the edge of the bed or examining table. If possible, the foot of the bed or table should be elevated. This position is particularly important if the patient is drowsy, since it will minimize the chances of aspiration. The tube should be passed gently, since no great force is necessary. If the patient can cooperate, have him or her swallow frequently; this permits the tube to move easily and rapidly.

If the catheter enters the larynx instead of the esophagus, dyspnea and severe coughing are produced; but these may be absent if the patient is deeply narcotized. If this occurs, the tube should be partially withdrawn before proceeding. If in doubt as to the placement of the tube, dip the free end in a glass of water. Continuous bubbling on expiration implies placement in the trachea, whereas gas from the stomach is usually expelled in two or three bursts. When the tube has reached the stomach, the glass syringe is then attached and the stomach contents are aspirated. In every instance, perform aspiration before installing a lavage solution.

Tap water is the fluid ordinarily used for lavage. However, increasing body fluid volume 5% with electrolyte-free water is enough to initiate the cardinal symptoms of water intoxication—tonic and clonic seizures with coma—which may appear without warning. Thus, it is far safer to substitute isotonic or one-half isotonic physiological saline solution for the tap water, particularly in children who have a limited tolerance for electrolyte depletion.

Stomach concretions from the massive ingestion of drugs (suicide attempts) and chemicals are a subtle problem in that many physicians are not alert to this possibility. A roentgenological flat plate of the abdomen will often be helpful in this diagnosis, although four pills often found in drug abuse emergencies are radio-opaque. These are: chloral hydrate, heavy metal, iron, and phenothiazine. More important, however, is an awareness of this possibility of stomach concretions in certain situations when the patient fails to respond to adequate therapy.

Castor oil as a solvent and agent to rush the material through the intestinal tract should be given whenever concretions are suspected.

Only small amounts of fluids should be installed at one time so that the passage of the drug into the upper intestinal tract will not be promoted. Repeat lavage ten or twelve times, or until the returns are clear. Save all washings; keep the first separate from the others for any analyses that might be indicated. Before the catheter is withdrawn, it should be pinched off or suction maintained to prevent aspiration.

A recently introduced device consisting of a double-lumen tube designed to deliver and aspirate simultaneously (or separately) allows the entire procedure of gastric lavage to be done in as little as 5 minutes.

REFERENCES

Kassirer, J. P. Serious acid-base disorders. *New England Journal of Medicine*, 1974, *291*, 773-776.

11
A Specific Approach to the Treatment of Drug and Alcohol Abusing Patients

OPIATE OVERDOSE

In recent years, overdose of narcotics has become a frequent problem in hospital emergency rooms. Many feel that uncomplicated opiate overdose induces a characteristic "shallow coma." The patient can be roused easily, but rapidly returns to coma, with respiratory rates of 4-6 per minute. Although narcotic overdose is usually accompanied by miosis, it should be noted that miosis also can be observed in severe barbiturate, ethanol, and phenothiazine overdose. Pupils may be dilated if hypoxia due to opiates is profound or if the overdose is from Demerol.

Treatment of opiate overdose involves the following procedures:

1. Clear airway, maintain respiration artificially, and administer oxygen.
2. Administer a narcotic antagonist, e.g., naloxone hydrochloride (Narcan) 0.4-0.8 mg I.V. (The pediatric dose is 0.01 mg/kg.) Naloxone is the drug of choice with a high margin of safety. In uncomplicated overdose, response to administration of antagonists is dramatic and diagnostic. Failure to see prompt improvement in respiratory rate implies that factors other than opiates are responsible for the respiratory depression that characterizes opiate overdose. The following considerations should be kept in mind when administering antagonists:
    a. Antagonists are effective for approximately 2 hours and re-

peat doses may be necessary. Heroin may remain active for 6 hours, methadone for 24-48 hours, and *l*-alpha-acetylmethadol (LAAM) for 48-72 hours, so care must be taken not to release the patient prematurely. As a rule of thumb, one should observe all opiate overdose cases for at least 12-24 hours at the hospital. Even after discharge, someone should be with the patient at all times for another 1-3 days. Therefore, the antagonist should be given at spaced intervals.
    b. In an active opiate dependent person, antagonists can precipitate a severe withdrawal syndrome.
    c. If respiratory depression has produced prolonged anoxia, the respirations may respond to naloxone but immediate return to a full conscious state may be delayed.
    d. When the pulmonary edema of opiate overdose is present, the administration of oxygen is the treatment of choice.
3. An occasional clinical problem may be caused by a medication error, e.g., a dose of 100 mg of methadone is administered to a patient taking 10 mg. If such errors are detected immediately after ingestion, i.e., the patient is alert and cooperative, Ipecac should be administered. As the interval increases between ingestion and detection of the error, the use of Ipecac has less benefit.

In general, patients should be normally active but under medical observation with naloxone close at hand. If doubt exists concerning the magnitude of the medication error, the patient must be observed closely and vital signs monitored at 15-minute intervals. Naloxone should be administered if somnolence or respiratory depression occur.

OPIATE WITHDRAWAL

The opiate withdrawal syndrome, while seldom fatal, can cause considerable discomfort and should be treated medically. The treatment of choice is to stabilize the patient on methadone and then to withdraw this drug gradually. The general principle in withdrawal is to provide the patient with sufficient drug to eliminate withdrawal signs without causing mental clouding or a "high." This is called "stabilizing" the patient. Once the patient is stabilized the dose of the stabilizing drug is decreased daily until the patient is drug free. *In all withdrawal attempts, constant clinical monitoring is necessary, since it is common for those dependent on heroin to be dependent also on sedatives or alcohol.*

For most patients addicted to "street" opiates where the actual dose is unknown, an initial methadone dose of 10-20 mg usually suppresses withdrawal signs. If 20 mg fails to suppress withdrawal symptoms, 5-10 mg increments may be given every 2 hours until the symptoms are suppressed. Then, the dose may be reduced approximately 5 mg/day until abstinence is achieved. Without coexisting major medical or psychiatric problems, detoxification from heroin can be achieved in 7-10 days, while detoxification from methadone may require more time, particularly if high doses were used. Studies of patients detoxifying from methadone maintenance indicate that very slow rates of detoxification are associated with higher retention rates in long-term addiction treatment.

Since those dependent upon heroin tend to be manipulative, more attention should be paid to objective withdrawal symptoms, e.g., lacrimation, rhinorrhea, pupillary dilation, and especially piloerection, than to subjective reports.

METHADONE WITHDRAWAL

Withdrawal of methadone in patients who have been maintained on this drug for years is presently an area of research. Methadone-maintained patients requesting to be withdrawn should be counseled and their motivations reviewed prior to any attempt to achieve abstinence. The abstinence attempt should occur at a time in which other areas of the patient's life are relatively free of stress. The attempt to achieve abstinence in methadone-maintained patients without supportive counseling has resulted in a return to street life and in some instances to death from heroin overdose.

The decision to attempt abstinence from methadone maintenance, then, is of serious import and should be approached carefully. Clinical experience indicates that slow reduction of methadone—5 mg per week at doses over 30-40 mg per day with decrements of 2-3 mg per week at lower doses—is associated with the best outcome. Withdrawal schedules should be individualized. Some patients may prefer to determine their own rate of withdrawal while others may prefer to have the physician determine the rate.

ALCOHOL OVERDOSE

Coma attributable to alcohol usually occurs in the young, first-exposure patient. It can also occur in adult patients, particularly binge drinkers who drink enormous quantities of alcohol rapidly. A mixture of drugs will commonly be found in association with the use of alcohol resulting in coma. It is important to obtain a blood/alcohol level and drug screen. There is usually a strong odor of alcohol about the patient. Respiratory depression can occur.

Because of the high incidence of pathological consequences of alcoholism, *always* look for other problems or causes of coma in the patient with alcohol odor. In particular, check for the following:

1. Hypoglycemia
2. Subdural hematoma
3. Trauma, including skull fracture
4. Septicemic meningitis
5. Cardiac arrhythmia (Ventricular fibrillation is a common cause of death; these patients should have cardiac monitoring.)
6. Wernicke's encephalopathy
7. Hepatic coma
8. Diabetic acidosis
9. Severe infectious process

Treatment of alcohol overdose involves the following procedures:

1. Nasogastric lavage should be performed within 1 hour of ingestion to remove any unabsorbed alcohol.
2. Give thiamine, 100 mg I.M. Glucose should be infused intravenously, as these patients may be hypoglycemic.
3. In the alcoholic presenting with coma, the probability of pneumonia is high. Therefore, a chest film and careful examination of the lungs is indicated.
4. The use of 10% or 40% fructose solutions to speed the metabolism of alcohol must be regarded as experimental at present. The danger of producing hyperuricemia or lactic acidosis is associated with the use of these fructose solutions.

ALCOHOL WITHDRAWAL

There are two factors which are useful in predicting the severity of the alcohol withdrawal syndrome. First is the drinking history, including the duration, amount, and pattern of drinking, and the degree of the development of alcohol tolerance. Second is the history of the signs and symptoms of physical dependence. While both are useful guides, the latter is the more useful of the two. For example, if a patient gives a history of early-morning shakiness and nausea that is relieved by alcohol, this suggests early physical dependence. Furthermore, the history of the type of withdrawal that the patient has had in the past can also give a clue to predicting the severity of the alcohol withdrawal syndrome under evaluation. If a patient has a history of delirium tremens (DT's) in the past, the physician should be alert to the likelihood of the repetition of this severe form of withdrawal. While alcohol withdrawal usually takes place upon cessation of drinking, it can also occur with reduced consumption of beverage alcohol and can also be precipitated by unrelated illnesses, particularly infectious disease.

Alcohol withdrawal can produce a variety of clinical syndromes from a mild hyperadrenergic state to hallucinosis and delirium. Many classification systems have evolved for the alcohol withdrawal syndrome. The terminology can be confusing, but what is clear is that there are mild and severe types of alcohol withdrawal, and there are some characteristics of withdrawal which may be associated with either the mild or the severe form.

The mild withdrawal syndrome is usually self-limited, physiologically resembling a hyperadrenergic state. Clinically there is anxiety, tremor of the outstretched hands or tongue, diaphoresis, tachycardia, systolic hypertension, nausea, vomiting, diarrhea, and sleep disturbances. It typically appears within 12-24 hours after the cessation of drinking, and its duration is usually 3-4 days.

The severe form of withdrawal, delirium tremens (DT's), is characterized by a symptom complex of profound confusion and disorientation, associated with hallucinations and autonomic and motor hyperactivity. It typically appears 3-4 days after the cessation of drinking, peaks on the fourth or fifth day, and then resolves in most patients over a subsequent 2-5 day period.

Alcoholic auditory hallucinosis is an unusual manifestation of alcohol withdrawal, clinically separate from the hallucinations of classical DT's. They occur unassociated with psychomotor agitation.

Rum fits are grand mal seizures occurring within 7-48 hours of cessation of drinking with the peak incidences at 24 hours. Fifty percent of the time they are single seizures. Only 3% become status epilepticus. Rum fits seldom occur after the onset of hallucinations or the delirium of DT's. If seizures are associated with delirium, other primary neurological or infectious disease etiologies must be ruled out.

While many sedative-hypnotic drugs have been used to treat the common abstinence syndrome, the benzodiazepines, chlordiazepoxide, and diazepam are currently the most widely used. The benzodiazepines have the advantage of being cross-tolerant with alcohol, and their long half-life is usually an advantage. Chlordiazepoxide (Librium) is the most widely used. In patients without severe and overt liver disease this drug is recommended.

For mild to moderate withdrawal, an initial test dose of 50-100 mg of chlordiazepoxide is given orally (P.O.) and the patient is observed 2-4 hours later. If the symptoms and signs of withdrawal are not ameliorated or are progressing, the dose is repeated. In most patients, an initial divided dose in the first 24-hour period from 50-200 mg usually provides mild sedation, decreases the tremulousness, and eases the bothersome symptoms of alcohol withdrawal. Occasionally, doses as high as 400-600 mg of chlordiazepoxide are necessary in the first 24 hours in severely tremulous and agitated patients. Because of the long half-life of this drug, subsequent daily doses can be reduced rapidly, usually by 50-100 mg a day. Thus, the usual pharmacotherapy for the alcohol withdrawal syndrome can be accomplished in 3-6 days. Benzodiazepines, particularly those with long half-lives, should be used with caution in elderly patients since such patients show increased sensitivity to the sedative effects of these drugs and also metabolize them more slowly. Severe hepatic disease can also complicate benzodiazepine therapy.

In patients with decompensating liver disease, lorazepam (Ativan) and oxazepam (Serax), both short-acting benzodiazepines, may be preferable. Lorazepam can be given 1-2 mg P.O. every 6-8 hours and oxazepam 15-30 mg P.O. every 6-8 hours.

When treating patients with delirium tremens, intravenous diazepam 10 mg initially followed by 5 mg every 5 minutes until a calming effect is achieved has proved to be effective. Intramuscular absorption of diazepam is less reliable. Patients may be switched from parenteral diazepam to oral diazepam or chlordiazepoxide as soon as they are able to tolerate oral medication. In addition to the use of benzodiazepines, the use of haloperidol, 2-4 mg intramuscularly every 2-6 hours as necessary, can be used as a supplement to diazepam in control of the agitation and is also helpful in controlling some of the behaviors secondary to hallucinations.

In addition to the use of these medications, the patient may require physical restraints. Careful monitoring of electrolyte balance and cardiac status is indicated. Particular attention should be given to the treatment of hypokalemia and hypomagnesemia as well as appropriate fluid and electrolyte replacement. Patients with DT's frequently have a coincident infectious disease, usually pneumonitis, which must be vigorously treated. The mortality rate rises sharply when DT's are accompanied by pneumonia, pancreatitis, or severe hepatitis.

While the severe forms of alcohol withdrawal require hospitalization and are a medical emergency, the mild syndrome need not be treated in a hospital setting. There are now a number of community-based detoxification centers which provide alcohol withdrawal treatment. Some employ pharmacological agents to aid in the detoxification. Others, called social setting or nonmedical detoxification centers, provide psychological and social support, usually in a home-like atmosphere designed to accomplish withdrawal without the use of pharmacological agents. These social-setting programs have been very effective in the treatment of the mild, self-limited form of alcohol withdrawal.

Detoxification from alcohol is not the treatment of alcoholism. It does provide an opportunity, however, to engage the alcoholic in the early stages of treatment. Every effort should be made to couple alcohol detoxification with referral to or the provision of continuing care for the chronic disease of alcoholism.

SEDATIVE-HYPNOTIC AND MINOR-TRANQUILIZER OVERDOSE

All central nervous system (CNS) depressants, if taken in sufficient quantity, appear to produce a similar comatose state, and CNS depressants are synergistic. Treatment is essentially symptomatic and medical in the acute phase. The following measures are involved:

1. Gastric lavage only if the drug was taken orally, recently, and the patient is conscious.

2. Respiratory support-intubation and mechanical assistance if necessary. Administer oxygen in high concentrations, ideally a tidal volume of 12-15 cc/kg body weight.
3. Treat shock with I.V. fluids and a vasopressor if indicated. Monitor electrolyte balance.
4. Continue monitoring of vital functions until consciousness returns. Treat cardiovascular problems symptomatically.
5. If barbiturates are implicated, diuresis and alkalinization of urine are helpful. Dialysis may be useful. Analeptic drugs are contraindicated.
6. Upon recovery, care must be taken with respect to possible suicide potential (CNS depressants are commonly used in suicide attempts) and possible addiction to CNS depressants.
7. Methaqualone overdose is reported to differ from barbiturate overdose in presenting with the gag reflex intact. Methaqualone does not depress the brain stem as do barbiturates. Intubation of such patients may be difficult because of this fact. Methaqualone overdose may present as delirium, restlessness, hypertonia, and convulsions. Dialysis may be helpful, but analgesics are contraindicated.
8. Glutethimide (Doriden) overdose may cause a cycle of coma and wakefulness as the drug is secreted into the gastrointestinal tract where it does not have effects and then is reabsorbed into the blood stream where once again it has CNS activity. As glutethimide is a fat soluble drug, gastric lavage, if performed, should be done with a 1:1 mixture of castor oil and water. Aqueous hemodialysis is less effective for glutethimide, and a dialysate of pure food-grade soybean oil is preferred.

SEDATIVE-HYPNOTIC AND MINOR-TRANQUILIZER WITHDRAWAL

Once a diagnosis of physical dependence on sedative-hypnotics is established, treatment for withdrawal becomes crucial. Because of the severity and even life-threatening nature of sedative-hypnotic withdrawal, close medical supervision of withdrawal is necessary. Withdrawal from barbiturates and other sedative-hypnotics generally should be accomplished in a hospital.

CNS depressants, including sedatives such as barbiturates, methaqualone, glutethimide, minor tranquilizers, and alcohol, are cross-tolerant, and theoretically withdrawal syndromes from them may be treated identically with any one of the groups of depressants. However, established practice in some treatment centers is that barbiturates are used for withdrawal from sedative-hypnotics, while a minor tranquilizer, such as chlordiazepoxide or diazepam, is used for alcohol or minor tranquilizer withdrawal. Given the demonstrated effectiveness of these approaches, there is no compelling rationale to change for those whose experience has been positive to such regimens.

The basic principle is to withdraw the individual slowly from sedative-hypnotic drugs. Careful monitoring of signs and symptoms is of utmost importance to assure a slow, gradual withdrawal. Adequate observation must be maintained to avoid the danger of seizures that may arise from a too rapid withdrawal. Treatment may be designed in accordance with either of two strategies: (a) slow withdrawal of the addicting agent or (b) substitution of a long-acting (phenobarbital) barbiturate and subsequent withdrawal of the substitute agent (Smith, 1976).

Traditionally, withdrawal from barbiturates is done with the addicting agent at dosages that produce mild intoxication. Generally, withdrawal should proceed at no greater than 100 mg of secobarbital or pentobarbital per day. Some clinicians use a pentobarbital challenge to help establish the degree of barbiturate tolerance and dependence when they initially see the patient. With this technique, 200 mg of a short-acting barbiturate such as pentobarbital are injected intramuscularly and the patient is observed before the next dose for toxicity to gauge true tolerance.

SUBSTITUTION TECHNIQUE

The rationale for substitution withdrawal is much the same as substituting methadone for heroin. The longer acting agent permits a withdrawal with fewer fluctuations in blood levels throughout the day, thereby allowing for the safe utilization of smaller dosages. Some clinicians prefer to substitute phenobarbital for the short-acting barbiturates or other sedative-hypnotic drugs and then withdraw the phenobarbital.

The safety factor for phenobarbital is greater than for the shorter acting barbiturates. Fatal amounts of phenobarbital are several times greater than toxic doses, and signs of toxicity produced by phenobarbital (such as sustained nystagmus, slurred speech, and ataxia) are easy to observe. Two days usually are required to transfer the individual from short-acting barbiturates to phenobarbital.

The dosage of phenobarbital is calculated by substituting one *sedative dose* (30 mg) of phenobarbital for each *hypnotic dose* (100 mg) of the short-acting barbiturate the patient reports using. In spite of the fact that many addicts exaggerate the magnitude of their addiction, the patient's history may be the best guide to initiating withdrawal. If the extent of the addiction has been grossly overstated, toxic symptoms will occur during the first day or so of treatment. This problem is easily managed by omitting one or more doses of phenobarbital and recalculating the daily dose. Should signs of withdrawal such as anxiety, sleep disturbances, orthostatic hypotension, hyperreflexia, muscle twitches, or stomach cramps occur, the total daily dose of phenobarbital is increased by approximately 25%. Should the patient show signs of phenobarbital toxicity (sustained nystagmus, slurred speech, or staggering gait), the daily dosage is reduced by 25% and withdrawal proceeds. The phenobarbital substitution technique may be used with short-acting sedative-hypnotics other than barbiturates. However, there is no reason to substitute with the benzodiazepines as their duration of action is similar to that of phenobarbital.

For patients dependent on benzodiazepines, detoxification using benzodiazepines is a gradual process usually taking several weeks. When the withdrawal is too abrupt seizures can occur, but unlike barbiturate addiction when seizures are seen early in withdrawal, the seizures in benzodiazepine withdrawal can occur days to weeks after abstinence is achieved.

OTHER TREATMENT APPROACHES

TRICYCLIC ANTIDEPRESSANT OVERDOSE

Tricyclic antidepressant overdose is characterized by coma, hyperpyrexia delirium, tachycardia, dry skin and mucous membranes, hypotension, and pupillary changes of either constriction or dilatation. Bladder distention, choreoathetosis, myoclonus, and arrhythmias may also occur. An increasing experience with tricyclic antidepressant overdose syndromes in both children and adults suggests that physostigmine salicylate (2 mg I.V.; pediatric dose 0.5 mg) therapy can be life-saving. Continuous monitoring of these cases is essential as fatal arrhythmias occur as a late complication (up to 5 days). Blood levels of those involved with tricyclic antidepressants may be low or not detectable because these drugs are bound to tissues and are only poorly bound to serum proteins. Effects of these drugs are sustained while the effects of anticholinesterase activity are short. Therefore, close clinical monitoring is mandatory. Anticholinergic agents such as glycopyrrolate (Robinul)(0.4-2.0 mg SC or I.V.) or propantheline bromide (Pro-Banthine)(15-30 mg I.M. or I.V.) may be necessary to correct the cholinergic effects of the physostigmine.

PENTAZOCINE ABUSE

Pentazocine (Talwin), an analgesic for mild to moderate degrees of pain, has been abused by an increasing number of people in the past decade. Talwin is taken orally, subcutaneously, or intravenously by abusers and is frequently mixed with tripelennamine (Pyribenzamine) and known as "T's and Blues." Infrequently, pentazocine is used with methylphenidate, Ritalin. Although pentazocine has mild narcotic antagonist properties and should cause narcotic withdrawal symptoms in active addicts, heroin users regularly report they use the drug when they cannot afford heroin, and that it relieves their narcotic withdrawal symptoms. They feel that they obtain relief and in some instances prefer pentazocine to heroin.

The mixture of pentazocine and tripelennamine, "T's and Blues," is reported to be like mixing heroin and cocaine, with pentazocine providing the narcotic high, and tripelennamine providing the stimulant high. Different ratios of pentazocine to tripelennamine are reported to yield different effects. A common ratio is two "T's" to one "Blue." Use of pentazocine and tripelennamine occasionally produces convulsions.

The dependence syndrome produced by pentazocine is usually mild and does not require treatment with decreasing doses of a narcotic drug such as methadone. In severe cases, some clinicians use low doses of methadone while others prefer to substitute decreasing doses of pentazocine. In most cases the nausea, restlessness, and insomnia will be well controlled with a few days of low-dose diazepam treatment.

In high doses pentazocine occasionally produces hallucinations and may produce an overdose syndrome of respiratory depression and coma which is responsive to naloxone.

Use of pentazocine parenterally causes severe sclerosis and ulceration of soft tissues. Treatment of the pentazocine user does not require use of narcotic maintenance, and general measures employed in treating other forms of "polydrug abuse" are applicable to pentazocine abusers.

PROPOXYPHENE ABUSE

Propoxyphene hydrochloride (Darvon), closely related chemically to methadone, is widely used to treat mild to moderate degrees of pain. Since it has a low degree of cross-tolerance to narcotics, it is not very effective in suppressing the opiate abstinence syndrome. Abuse of propoxyphene occurs, and the clinician may encounter overdoses which are characterized by respiratory depression, miosis, and coma but also, on occasion, by focal and generalized seizures, pulmonary edema, and/or cardiac arrhythmias.

Propoxyphene has been implicated in an increasing number of overdose deaths in the United States in the past decade. In three-quarters of these deaths multiple drugs have been ingested. Many of these deaths appear to be associated with suicide attempts.

Repeated use of Darvon is associated with tolerance and physical dependence. High doses (over 600 mg) sometimes cause hallucinations. The withdrawal syndrome is usually a mild version of the opiate abstinence syndrome and may be treated without substitution of any drugs. Sedatives and/or anxiolytics for a few days may be useful in treating this withdrawal syndrome. If withdrawal is severe, propoxyphene or low doses of methadone may have to be substituted for a 5-10 day period. Prescription of large amounts of propoxyphene, especially to emotionally disturbed and/or suspected drug and alcohol abusers, should be avoided.

ABUSE OF VOLATILES

This class of drugs includes glue, lacquers, enamel, brake fluids, lighter fluid, gasoline, aerosols, paint thinner, nitrous oxide, amyl and butyl nitrite, and other agents.

Volatiles do not usually cause coma, because it is easy to titrate the dose used to get high ("huffing"); but coma can occur if the person falls on the rag saturated with the material.

Mucosal blisters in the mouth or nose, or the odor of the inhalant on breath are the only helpful physical signs. Therefore, obtaining historical information is important.

Respiratory depression is possible. The cardiovascular system should be monitored closely. Ventricular fibrillation and other arrhythmias have been observed in users of volatiles. Over 100 sudden deaths a year are reported in the United States associated with volatiles. Many of these deaths are attributable to cardiac arrhythmias.

Neurological examination of such cases should be extensive. Peripheral neuropathies and severe neurological syndromes have been observed occasionally in solvent abusers. Industrial workers may also present with neuropathies in association with working conditions or in association with abuse patterns. Hepatic, renal, and bone marrow function can be severely affected by the use of volatiles. Families of patients involved with volatiles should be advised that complications may develop 24 hours or more after use. Therefore, they should bring the patient back to the hospital if symptoms occur.

STIMULANT ABUSE

Stimulants, including many amphetamine derivatives, phenmetrazine (Preludin), methylphenidate, cocaine, and others, are more widely abused than generally recognized. In view of their substantial danger of abuse, medically approved stimulants should be prescribed carefully and only when the benefits exceed the potential dangers implicit in these drugs. When grossly abused, all stimulants produce a similar clinical picture, including some or all of the following signs and symptoms:

1. Insomnia
2. Anorexia, with possible malnutrition
3. Hypertension, tachycardia, elevated body temperature
4. Dilated pupils
5. Muscular tremor
6. Possible damage to nasal mucosa (if taken as snuff); extensive needle scars and associated pathology (if taken intravenously)
7. Verbosity—constant "rambling" talk
8. Impulsivity

9. Extreme nervousness, suspiciousness, and hostility that may develop into a characteristic stimulant-induced paranoid psychosis. This psychosis is very similar to that of paranoid schizophrenia, but the short-term prognosis is good. With abstinence from the drug, psychotic manifestations usually disappear within a few days, although occasionally they may last for several weeks or months. The latter should be treated with Haldol.

ACUTE OVERDOSE

This condition is rather uncommon with most stimulants and is seen mainly in cocaine abuse. It can include severe hyperthermia, convulsions, cerebrovascular accidents, and possible cardiovascular or respiratory collapse. Treatment must be rapid and appropriate to the symptomatology, including respiratory or cardiac support if indicated, sedation, and aggressive treatment of hyperthermia. Acidification of the urine with ammonium chloride, 12 g/day P.O. or I.V., significantly enhances amphetamine excretion.

CHRONIC ABUSE SYNDROME

Treatment is primarily psychotherapeutic. In severe psychotic reactions, short-term psychiatric hospitalization may be indicated. Minor tranquilizers will control anxiety. Davis, Sekerke, and Janowski (1973) recommend that haloperidol may alleviate psychotic symptomatology. Phenothiazines are not indicated as they retard the excretion of amphetamines.

STIMULANT WITHDRAWAL

Usually the chronic abuse syndrome will be alleviated after a single sleep period (often 24-48 hours long). However, possibly due either to depletion of brain catecholamines or other causes, there will usually be a withdrawal syndrome that may need additional treatment. This syndrome, which may last for weeks or months, is characterized by:

1. Moderate to severe depression, with possible suicidal ideation
2. Sleep disturbances, lethargy

3. Postpsychotic suspiciousness or hostility
4. Mild tremor in extremities, various aches and pains

Initially, treatment should be oriented to restoration of biological health including nondependency-producing sedatives at night until a regular sleep cycle is restored; major tranquilizers only if psychosis persists; ample diet, including vitamin supplement; and treatment of associated pathology, e.g., hepatitis. Antidepressants should be used cautiously during the first week of treatment, as blood levels of stimulants may persist for some time, a situation that creates the possibility of undesirable interaction between the two classes of drugs. They are needed for severe depressive reactions, however. After medical needs are met, there should be referral for long-term care.

HALLUCINOGENS

Hallucinogens are widely available and subject to frequent experimentation. Due to the variety of hallucinogens and the unpredictable content of illicit drugs, the abuser frequently does not know what he or she ingested.

CLINICAL SIGNS

Patients who seek medical attention after using hallucinogenic chemicals may be disoriented, anxious, or panicky. They may have sensory disturbances including abnormal sensitivity to or interpretation of stimuli. Hallucinations, of course, can be prominent. There may also be ideas of reference and inappropriate affect.

Psychiatric syndromes resulting from hallucinogens can, at times, be distinguished from ordinary psychotic states by the history of drug use, by the presence of time-sense distortions, and by the relative preponderance of visual phenomena in the drug-related emergency. In addition, the physician will sense that defense mechanisms are not damaged to the degree seen in the acute schizophrenic break. Patients on a "bad trip" are more likely to report that they see or hear "crazy" things, and their judgment and control appear to be more intact than in the case of the acute psychotic break. In addition, the symptomatology of the "bad trip" tends to be labile: delusional symptoms are transient, affect changes rapidly. Often the patient can emerge suddenly from extreme confusion to complete rationality, only to return to confusion minutes later. Physiological signs, such as dilated pupils, cramps, nausea, or mild tachycardia, are common.

Most individuals who have used hallucinogens report difficulty talking or communicating while intoxicated. Nor is it surprising that many become frightened. Hallucinogens do not usually leave significant long-term pathology, but flashbacks and chronic psychosis have been reported. Although differing somewhat from drug to drug, most hallucinogens begin taking effect 1-2 hours after an oral dose. Dimethyltryptamine produces effects in 15-30 minutes. Intoxication usually lasts for less than 5 hours, then declines over the next 8 hours. The individual can be expected to be "normal" after 24 hours, although he or she may report unusual thoughts or feelings as much as a week later. The most common adverse reaction is panic, usually because the psychological factors involved in the use of the drug are pathological and because the social setting is not supportive.

The relatively rare serious physical reaction may consist of convulsions, elevated body temperature, hypertension, severe vomiting, respiratory depression, nystagmus, and/or cardiac dysfunction. Such disorders may be caused by PCP or belladonna alkaloids (Jimson weed).

FLASHBACKS

Flashbacks develop in a small percentage of hallucinogenic experiences. Typically these are recurrent "spells" of a few seconds or minutes of acute depersonalization or hallucinosis, or they may take the form of a somatic delusion. Usually they are reminiscent of the hallucinogenic experience. They are often precipitated by fatigue or acute stress and could persist for many weeks. They ordinarily stop permanently after a few months, and reassurance is usually adequate treatment. In more severe cases, minor tranquilizers or psychotherapy may be indicated.

TREATMENT FOR HALLUCINOGEN INTOXICATION

The following approach to hallucinogen intoxication treatment is useful in most situations. However, the management of PCP intoxication is an important exception and will be discussed separately.

Treatment must be performed in a nonthreatening fashion. After checking vital signs to eliminate the possibility of physiological danger, the patient should be "talked down" or "brought down," i.e., treated in a place that is quiet and dimly lit. Low levels of sensory input are desirable because of the distractability involved.

If a reliable friend of the patient is available, it is usually wise to keep him or her present, but only a small number of people should be involved. Emphasis should be on alleviating anxiety. Simple direct communications are helpful. ("Everything's going to be fine," "The drug will wear off in a few hours," "Are you feeling better now?" etc.) Such simplicity and directness should be coupled with friendliness and assistance in orientation. ("You're in a hospital," "You took a pill," "Would you like some orange juice?") Quiet music, or even television, can be useful. At least one person should remain with the patient until the effects of the drug have worn off. If the patient keeps his or her eyes open, the reaction will be less intense.

Chemotherapy should be reserved for refractory cases whose agitation is not reduced by psychological approaches. In such instances, chlordiazepoxide or diazepam can be helpful. Phenothiazines should not be used since they may interact with many hallucinogenic drugs to cause lability of blood pressure and/or worsening of the psychotic-like state. In some cases, short-term or long-term hospitalization may be necessary.

PHENCYCLIDINE (PCP) REACTIONS

At present, PCP is frequently a cause of many emergency problems. PCP is a drug often sold under other names. It is usually sold as THC (tetrahydrocannabinol), the "essence" of pot. Depending on dose and route of administration, different syndromes can be observed. In addition, since PCP is frequently manufactured by illegal and sometimes amateur chemists, it may not be pure. One possible contaminant is a synthetic intermediate (PCC) which contains an organic group which will decompose to yield hydrogen cyanide. Thus cyanide poisoning may accompany PCP overdose and psychosis. Bloody vomiting in a PCP user should suggest the possibility that a contaminant is present.

A patient who is not tolerant to PCP and has taken low doses (5-10 mg) of the drug may present with intoxication and agitation. The latter can be severe and violent behavior may result. Higher doses produce motor inhibition, and catatonic-like states are seen. Typically, the patient exhibits a blank stare and sits or lies motionless. Gait ataxia is prominent, and horizontal and vertical nystagmus may be present. Pulse and blood pressure, both systolic and diastolic, are elevated. Analgesia, muscle rigidity, and amnesia are common.

As the dose increases—in the 10-30 mg range the patient may become stuporous or frankly comatose. In coma, the patient's eyes may remain open. Vomiting and hypersalivation may be present. At high doses (50-100 mg) patients may have seizures, opisthotonos, increased deep tendon reflexes (DTR), and have Cheyne Stokes respirations or apnea. Testing procedures are available in laboratories for the detection of PCP in the urine. When PCP has been used in high doses, it can also be detected in the blood.

The low-dose state is frequently interpreted as secondary to an unknown psychedelic drug. The absence of mydriasis and the presence of gait ataxia, hypertension, and horizontal and vertical nystagmus are diagnostic of a PCP intoxication. The key to management of the low-dose acute intoxicated state is sensory reduction with observation at a distance. Exacerbation of clinical symptoms is seen even with minimal verbal or physical stimulation. The patient should be placed on a cushioned surface of the floor in a quiet room. Someone should be present to monitor the patient's condition. Protection from self-harm may also be necessary. Clinicians prefer the use of haloperidol or diazepam to control the sometimes widely fluctuating behavior of the patient who has taken PCP.

A moderate dose of PCP may be initially interpreted as a sedative-hypnotic overdose. The presence of hypertension and hyperreflexia (DTR) and the absence of prominent respiratory depression differentiate the PCP-intoxicated state from sedative-hypnotic overdose. In a patient who presents with the moderate-dose state, blood pressure should be monitored and close observation maintained for clonic movements indicative of the muscle rigidity that usually precedes seizure activity. Again, sensory stimulation should be controlled and minimized. Gastric lavage is indicated in view of the large quantities of PCP that have been recovered from the gastric contents in fatal cases of intoxication.

Cases involving ingestion of high doses of PCP that present as undiagnosed coma may be difficult to differentiate from other causes. Again, if hypertension is evident and there is no significant depression of respiration, sedative-hypnotic overdose can be ruled out. If, in addition, opisthotonic posturing is present in a child or seizure activity is present in an adult, a PCP intoxication should be suspected in addition to various neurological syndromes. The characteristic prolonged recovery phase lasting several days to a week is diagnostic of PCP intoxication.

If status epilepticus develops, judicious administration of diazepam (Valium) in 2-3 mg increments I.V. is indicated. Respirations should be monitored closely following the administration of diazepam. Some barbiturates act synergistically with phencyclidine to depress respiration. The use of barbiturates to treat convulsions or status epilepticus therefore is contraindicated.

Hypertension is a common finding in high-dose PCP intoxication. If this condition persists, it can be life-threatening due to intravenous bleeding. Diazoxide has been reported to be effective in lowering blood pressure during a hypertensive crisis thought to be secondary to PCP.

The high-dose intoxicated patient may remain comatose for a period of 12 hours or more (Aronow & Done, 1978). The principles of sensory isolation and protection from self-harm apply to the prolonged recovery period that may last several days and may require admission to a psychiatric unit. Death in PCP coma has occurred.

One important advance in the treatment of PCP intoxication is the finding that the acidification of the urine markedly enhances PCP excretion, thereby shortening the duration of the adverse reaction to PCP. This can be administered by the intravenous or nasogastric route. Patients who are candidates for acidification should have adequate renal and hepatic function. Ammonium chloride is administered via nasogastric tube. Vitamin C and cranberry juice are given orally to assist in acidification of urine to a pH of 5.

Since PCP is a weakly basic, it ionizes in acid media. Some investigators believe that PCP ionizes in gastric contents thus removing PCP from the blood by back diffusion into the gastrointestinal tract. For this reason, another therapeutic measure to enhance PCP removal is continuous or intermittent gastric suction. Also, as the gastric contents travel down the gastrointestinal tract they become alkaline; PCP then diffuses back into the blood stream with associated effects on the brain and behavior. This sequence may account for the clinical observations of normal behaviors interspersed with irrational behaviors in PCP users.

Prolonged psychotic reactions following PCP ingestion have been observed. Associated severe anxiety, bizarre behavior, disorientation, "awake coma," and violence may present difficult clinical problems. Chronic psychosis following PCP ingestion should be treated with measures commonly employed in treating psychoses from other causes. Phenothiazines should be avoided in acute phase PCP reactions because of the possibility of inducing hypertensive crisis or hypotensive episodes. Protecting the patient and those about him or her is a major concern.

CANNABIS

In the doses currently available in the United States, cannabis use is infrequently associated with reactions severe enough to require medical attention. Occasionally acute panic will develop and in such cases the general measures of "talking down" described above should be instituted. Cannabis use, particularly in the instance of hashish and hash oil (forms of cannabis with much higher potency), can be associated with psychotic behavior. In such cases current knowledge suggests that treatment should be oriented to underlying personal problems, not to the drug per se. Tennant's (1972) experience among United States soldiers in Germany suggests that at very high doses behavioral problems are varied, severe, and frequent. But evidence on this point is conflicting. Rubin and Comitas (1975) studied 30 adult Jamaicans who used ganja, a potent form of cannabis. In comparison to a control group of 30 Jamaicans who did not use cannabis products, the users of ganja differed only in having hematologic changes attributable to a relative hypoxemia. The hypoxemia was, in the opinion of Rubin and Comitas, attributable to the fact that ganja is smoked along with tobacco. Rubin and Comitas did not observe behavioral problems that discriminated between groups. Mehndiratta and Wig (1975), however, studied heavy users of cannabis in India and found that heavy users of cannabis products did differ from controls in having more pulmonary complaints, a poorer nutritional state, more anemia, poorer work records, and more frequent occurrence of behavioral problems. The issue of loss of motivation in young people is a concern of some researchers and clinicians.

Recent data indicate that cannabis is not the safe drug it was assumed to be just a few years ago. Studies of pulmonary function in relatively low-dose cannabis users indicate that smoking this substance is associated with the same kinds of pulmonary pathology observed in tobacco smokers. Cannabis use appears to inhibit ovulation in human females and to be associated with low sperm counts, abnormal motility patterns, and abnormal sperm forms in human males. Recent research also indicates that during cannabis intoxication, psychomotor coordination is affected adversely, thus making it difficult to operate an automobile or a machine safely. Other questions concerning the effect of cannabis on the immune mechanism and on subcortical brain centers are being pursued by a variety of investigators.

MULTIPLE DRUG ABUSE

Multiple drug abuse is quite common. The use of barbiturates to "smooth" an amphetamine trip, or the use of alcohol to heighten hallucinogen effects are examples. There are no specific physical signs. Knowledge of the pharmacology of drug interactions may be important to the acute treatment of such patients.

Studies have shown that a higher incidence of psychopathology is found among polydrug abusers than in those individuals abusing a single substance such as heroin or alcohol. This has contributed to much confusion among clinicians involved in the detoxification of clients because the psychological symptoms that have been ascribed to drug abuse actually became worse when the clients were drug free. The clinicians failed to appreciate the significance of clients using a drug of abuse to self-medicate underlying psychiatric disorders. Consequently, the failure to recognize the high degree of psychopathology among the polydrug user population has led to a striking record of treatment failure within traditional health care systems, including drug treatment programs.

In the instance of multiple dependencies, the safest technique appears to be to withdraw one drug at a time, while stabilizing the patient on whatever other drugs he or she may be dependent. For example, if the patient depends on heroin and barbiturates, the patient is stabilized with methadone while decreasing doses of barbiturates are given for the detoxification of barbiturate dependence. Once the barbiturates are completely withdrawn, methadone doses can be subsequently reduced.

REFERENCES

Aronow, R., & Done, A. K. Phencyclidine overdose: An emerging concept of management. *JACEP,* 1978, 7, 56-59.

Davis, J., Sekerke, J., & Janowski, D. Drug interactions involving drugs of abuse. In National Commission on Marijuana and Drug Use, *Drug use in America: Problem in perspective* (Second report of the National Commission on Marijuana and Drug Use). Washington, D.C.: U.S. Government Printing Office, 1973.

Mehndiratta, S. S., & Wig, N. N. Psycho-social effects of long term cannabis use in India. *Drug and Alcohol Dependence,* 1975, *1*, 71-82.

Rubin, V., & Comitas, L. *Ganja in Jamaica.* Paris: Mouton, 1975.

Smith, D. E. *Polydrug abuse and comprehensive treatment intervention.* Rockville, Maryland: National Clearinghouse for Drug Abuse Information, 1976.

Tennant, F. S., Jr. Drug abuse in the US Army, Europe. *Journal of the American Medical Association,* 1972, *221,* 1146-1149.

12
Drug and Alcohol-Related Problems in the Physician's Office

Physicians may be asked for information and guidance on drug- and alcohol-related problems by parents or by adolescents. Frequently parents need to turn to someone when they suspect or know that their children are using drugs. The key concepts in responding to such requests are to try to clarify what questions are being asked and to determine the significance of drugs in the young person's total adaptation.

Parents and teenagers alike frequently will not be clear on what information they want because they are expressing a concern or a fear that is not explicit. "My son/daughter is using marijuana. Will he or she become a drug addict?" represents a type of question commonly posed. This question expresses a fear, or a number of fears, as much as or more than a request for information. If the physician responds with comments and questions that assist in clarifying these fears, he or she will be of much greater assistance than if he or she answers "Yes/No, your son/daughter probably will/won't become a drug addict." Such an answer causes closure and does not allow the parents to develop an understanding of what information they want.

The physician should ask questions that elicit information. For example, "How do you know that your son or daughter is using marijuana?" or "Who does he or she use it with? Where? How often?" The physician should try to elicit sufficient detail to permit an understanding of the relative importance of the drug- or alcohol-using behavior in the adolescent's life. If a young person is doing well in school, participating in age-appropriate activities, e.g., band, sports, clubs, etc., and is generally adapting satisfactorily, the physician may conclude that the parent has a normal young person who is experimenting with marijuana and/or alcohol in response to the pressures of modern youth culture. This young person may be behaving exactly as his or her parents did with respect to alcohol when they were teenagers.

On the opposite end of the clinical spectrum, the physician may elicit data indicating a seriously disturbed young person with a major drug problem—such as dependence on opioids, CNS depressants, or alcohol. In this event, the physician will be able to assist in proportion to his or her knowledge of treatment resources. In any event, the physician should communicate clearly to the parent an intention to follow the situation. Creating a feeling of support and continuity of support can be of great importance to both the family and the youth in trouble.

Teenagers may turn to a physician for advice on drug- or alcohol-related matters. Frequently teenagers will not be able to ask for help directly, but will need to talk about some abstract state that is troublesome for them, e.g., "What can a bad trip do to you?" etc. The physician should respect the patient's need in this regard and discuss the state or condition until such time as he or she feels comfortable in identifying the locus of the problem. The physician usually will not be able to attribute the problem to the teenager directly if the teenager is moderately or severely disturbed. The physician should pledge confidentiality if that is what the young person wants. Many states have laws that support specifically the right of a physician to treat a minor without notifying the parents. Teenagers, in fact, may need someone with whom to discuss their parents.

Currently, laws forbid physicians from giving drugs to narcotic addicts to support their habits unless the patient is in a hospital being treated for a medical, surgical, or obstetric problem. Physicians are permitted to prescribe opioid drugs in whatever quantities, and for whatever period they deem advisable, when opioid-dependent patients are being treated in a hospital for conditions other than their opioid dependence. The basic office service that the physician should offer to the opioid dependent patient is diagnosis and referral. In office settings, the principal problem in diagnosis may be simply a low index of suspicion. As drug problems have spread into the middle class, however, the likelihood has increased substantially of encountering opioid dependent persons in routine office practice.

A supply of naloxone should be kept in the office emergency kit to administer to the opioid-overdose patient who may be present in an office setting.

The physician should be aware of the problem of status inversion that may complicate his or her relationship with opioid dependent patients. The opioid dependent person is likely to view the physician as potentially manipulative and dishonest as the addict is himself or herself. This view is generated, in part, by the rejection of the establishment implicit in the drug-using culture, and in part by the discrimination against drug dependent persons that occurs in our medical care systems. Shorn of status and subject to careful scrutiny by the addict, who usually seeks to manipulate him or her, the physician may experience problems in knowing how to respond. If the physician seeks to learn about the addict and the addict's world, and if the physician adheres to his or her ideal of service, he or she will navigate these difficult straits.

The physician should resist the temptation to give narcotics for maintenance of the addiction under the guise of some indistinct need for analgesia. In almost every instance, the physician will be manipulated; the addict will sell his or her medicine, and the physician will only be serving as a supplier of illicit narcotics to the street.

Obviously, the better informed the physician is on drug and alcohol matters the better counselor he or she will be. The National Clearinghouse for Drug Abuse Information and The National Clearinghouse for Alcohol Information are excellent resources for the physician. From these sources the physician can obtain excellent, up-to-date reviews of specific drugs.

The materials available from these sources are printed at cost and, therefore, are not a drain on the physician's book and journal budget. Many consultations with both parents and teenagers can be conducted satisfactorily by referring to these sources. The physician should be aware that most drug- and alcohol-related consultations are requests for information, not requests for therapy. In counseling drug and alcohol abusers, the physician also will do well to learn about drug and alcohol treatment efforts in his or her community. Although the stereotypical "street" attitude among young people is that one does not ask doctors questions about drugs or anything else, the physician who is willing and able to assist in counseling on drug- or alcohol-related problems will be able to serve. Drug abusers will respond to good service regardless of who renders it.

Each state has a Single State Agency that can assist the physician with a listing of drug and alcohol treatment centers.

In the event that the addict is genuinely seeking help, the physician may use monographs from the sources cited to learn about treatment possibilities. The physician can refer the addict to the Single State Agency to identify the local possibilities.

The physician also should learn about the growing numbers of programs aimed at assisting the impaired physician. This is a problem that will involve physicians increasingly in coming years. Many state medical societies have a panel of physicians who will respond to physicians in trouble with substance abuse. References in the bibliography will provide the interested reader with detailed descriptions of various state programs and with concrete referral sources.

Poor history taking, inadequate primary and continuing medical education, and stereotyping of alcoholics as morally inadequate combine to make alcoholism the most frequently missed diagnosis in medical practice. It is probable that the frequency of alcoholics in general medical practice is 5-10%. Some experts estimate that 15-20% of all hospital beds in the country are devoted to problems caused by alcohol.

The most important first step for a physician is to realize that he or she can offer meaningful assistance to people with alcohol-related problems. There are a number of important elements:

1. Increase the index of suspicion—suspect alcoholism in everyone. Alcoholism occurs in every social strata, ethnic, and social group, both sexes, and increasingly at younger ages.
2. Ask about it and/or use simple office screening tests such as the Michigan Alcoholism Screening Test (MAST). Although denial is common among alcohol abusers, on occasion the act of asking will elicit a response of concern about the problem. No matter what the habit, people are ambivalent about it. People who smoke, drink, eat too much, or take drugs are concerned about it. You owe them the question: "Do you worry about your habits/drinking/smoking?"
3. If your best judgment is that your patient is abusing alcohol, you must present this judgment to the patient. The technique is called confrontation, but as used technically this term implies confrontation with concern and with an absence of moral judgment, as contrasted to the lay meaning of the term confrontation which implies harshness. No matter how vigorous the denial, it is important to present your judgment. Tell the patient that failure to recognize and change a pattern of pathological drinking may lead to serious medical and/or psychiatric problems.
4. Recommend Alcoholics Anonymous (AA). Your management

of an alcoholic requires a program which has many elements. Perhaps the most important is to use AA. Part of your preparation for treating alcoholics and for learning about alcohol is to attend AA meetings. Then you will know how well AA groups in your community fit the needs of a particular patient, and your education concerning alcoholism will be expanded.

5. Involve the family. The most constant characteristic of the alcoholic patient is psychological isolation from those close to him or her. Confidentiality laws make it impossible to communicate your clinical findings concerning an alcoholic patient if the patient does not wish this. But many patients will consent to bringing in the spouse. Once this has been accomplished you may wish to use Al-Anon or Alateen as part of your management program.

6. Change the pattern. Frequently this will require hospitalization to break up the pattern of regular heavy drinking so that the patient may begin to think in an organized way about the future. If hospitalization is not necessary or feasible try to influence the patient to break up pathological social networks that reinforce drinking behavior; or, conversely, the alcoholic who has become a social isolate should be urged to establish new social contacts free of pressure to drink. The basic principle is to put people back into the life of the alcoholic while getting the alcohol out. This will require a thorough review of the fabric of the alcoholic's life.

7. Consider using Antabuse. See Chapter 14 for technical details.

8. Be careful of sedative-hypnotics. Alcoholics and alcohol abusing individuals commonly have problems with anxiety/depression feeling states and with insomnia. It is important to point out that with continued sobriety from all psychoactive substances, these states will resolve. Of course, if there is question of a psychiatric disorder, psychiatric consultation should be obtained. People with major affective disorders may abuse alcohol and will need lithium or antidepressant drugs if they are to maintain themselves. The long-term use of sedative-hypnotics and/or minor tranquilizers is to be avoided.

9. Project a feeling of confidence. Almost universally the alcohol abusing person feels hopeless to change. An untutored physician may reinforce this feeling and thereby seal off any real possibility for recovery. After some exposure to problems related to al-

cohol abuse, the physician should be able to develop real confidence. There are no higher rewards in medicine than in seeing a family reintegrated after one of its members has been involved with alcohol.

The same principles discussed above can be applied to the growing number of abusers of "polydrugs," i.e., benzodiazepines, marijuana, chloral hydrate, ethchlorvynol, glutethimide, methaqualone, etc. Indeed, the drug culture has succeeded in adding these drugs to our national alcohol problems. Consumption of alcohol, particularly among our young, has increased along with the use of the many classes of drugs which have come into vogue in the past decade.

The physician should recognize that persistent history taking may be required because frequently users of these substances will not realize that they have dependence-producing potential. Benzodiazepines are a case in point; it is recognized that moderate doses, close to doses in the therapeutic range, may produce at least mild dependence. Close monitoring for signs of withdrawal and, in particular, for seizures is necessary in the early stages of treatment. Withdrawal from diazepam may not occur for 7-10 days following cessation of intake. Thus, the index of suspicion has to be high and sustained.

13
Management of Opiate Dependent Patients in the General Hospital

The physician will encounter three types of opiate dependent patients on general medical wards: (1) the patient who is enrolled in a bona fide methadone maintenance program, (2) the "street addict" who states or demonstrates that he or she is dependent on heroin, but who is not in treatment for his or her dependency, and (3) those who have become narcotic dependent in connection with their medical-surgical treatment.

METHADONE MAINTENANCE PATIENTS ON THE GENERAL MEDICAL WARD

For patients who state that they are enrolled in a methadone maintenance program, prompt communication with the program physician or the patient's counselor is necessary to confirm the fact of enrollment and to learn the maintenance dose of methadone. In addition, information can be obtained regarding special medical or psychosocial problems encountered during the opiate dependent person's course of treatment. Physicians should be aware that those dependent on opiates have a tendency to exaggerate their needs; before the clinician initiates treatment with methadone, the maintenance dose should be confirmed. An inexperienced physician occasionally will make a decision to administer methadone to the maintained patient without consulting the treatment program. This lack of communication may result in giving the patient an inadvertent methadone overdose. After confirming the dose the physician should not change it, nor should he or she attempt to detoxify the patient. It is important that no attempt be made by the hospital physician to alter the treatment for drug dependency in a patient enrolled in a maintenance program.

Methadone maintained patients enrolled in a drug abuse program are best managed by continuing methadone at the usual maintenance levels with once-a-day oral administration. If oral administration is not possible, intramuscular or subcutaneous administration of methadone will suffice. A regimen in which methadone is given parenterally in 5-10 mg doses every 8 hours will cover most cases. It is rare that this parenteral dose level will have to be increased, regardless of the preadmission oral methadone-maintenance dose. An alternate regimen consists of giving two-thirds of the maintenance dose in two equally divided doses, 12 hours apart. For example, a patient maintained on 100 mg per day of methadone would receive 35 mg of methadone parenterally every 12 hours as long as he or she must remain NPO. A methadone-maintained patient who is placed NPO for a surgical or diagnostic procedure must be given some narcotic on the day of the procedure and for as long as oral feedings are precluded. Full doses of oral methadone should be reinstituted when oral fluids are well tolerated.

Continued contact with the patient's maintenance program is an important part of the management of the hospitalized drug dependent patient. Management of hostile behavior, of family problems, of visitors who are unruly or involved in the selling or taking of drugs, and the making of discharge plans will be facilitated by communicating frequently with the staff of the patient's treatment program.

Stabilization with methadone can be safely continued as long as the patient is ill. Studies of patients in maintenance treatment for heroin dependency who have been stabilized with methadone in high doses for 3 or more years have revealed minimal side effects and no toxic effects. Undesired effects include increased sweating, persistent constipation, urinary retention, and drowsiness if the dose is excessive. Abnormal liver function and serum protein tests are reported in 75-90% of heroin dependent patients entering the hospital or treatment programs, probably as a result of repeated use of unsterile needles, injection of foreign substances, and excessive use of ethanol. These abnormalities persist without significant change during methadone-maintenance treatment.

Upon discharge, it is important that the patient return to his program at once for continuation of maintenance treatment. It is undesirable and illegal for the hospital physician to undertake maintenance responsibility for an outpatient.

"STREET ADDICTS" ON THE GENERAL MEDICAL WARD

"Street addicts," i.e., patients who state or demonstrate that they are dependent on narcotics but who are not enrolled in a drug abuse program, present a different problem. The first principle of managing such patients is to support and to continue their addiction to opiates until the acute phase of their illness is over. This can be achieved by placing them on methadone. Treatment is compromised if patients have to suffer concurrently from opiate withdrawal and the distress associated with illness, trauma, or labor.

Attempts to withdraw patients from opiates during an acute medical or surgical crisis will complicate the management of such crises and are unlikely to be successful in achieving abstinence from opiates. Therefore, decisions about withdrawal from opiates should be deferred until the acute phase of the patient's illness is over.

Because the drug dependent patient's history cannot be relied upon and because symptoms are sometimes feigned or exaggerated, the American Psychiatric Association Task Force on Drug Dependence (1971) recommends that methadone be given to "street addicts" only after the appearance of physical signs of the abstinence syndrome. It should be noted that the use of a narcotic drug, even if periodic, cannot be equated with narcotic dependency. Care must be exercised in initiating methadone treatment to avoid causing dependency on methadone in a person who is not already dependent upon narcotic drugs. The clinician must make repeated evaluations for withdrawal signs and symptoms during the first 24-36 hours of hospitalization. In selected patients, the clinician may conclude that the presence of fresh "needle tracks" and a positive admission urine test for morphine or quinine are sufficient evidence to begin treatment with a modest dose (10 mg per day) of methadone or a short-acting narcotic to forestall withdrawal. Exceptional circumstances may occur in which intense subjective complaints in a known drug-dependent person can be treated with a small dose of methadone (5 mg per day).

Heroin (diacetylmorphine) is seldom detected as such in the urine of heroin dependent patients because it is deacetylated rapidly. Heroin appears in the urine as morphine, which may be present for 12-24 hours following last use of heroin. Because quinine is used to cut street heroin, it is found frequently in the urine of heroin dependent persons and can be detected for 5-10 days after the use of "street" heroin.

Based on the physical examination, opiate withdrawal signs and symptoms can be classified according to severity (Fultz & Senay, 1975). As noted in Table 13-1, the initial dose of methadone should be: Grade 1 = 5 mg; Grade 2 = 10 mg; Grade 3 = 15 mg; and Grade 4 = 20 mg. Supplementary doses of 5-10 mg of methadone may be provided if withdrawal signs are not suppressed or as signs reappear.

A short-acting narcotic such as morphine or dihydromorphinone (Dilaudid) used in a small dose may be preferable to the long-acting methadone for initial treatment if the diagnosis of physical dependency is in doubt. Also, short-acting narcotics may be needed as additional treatment agents even if there is no question of the presence of addic-

Table 13-1
RELATION BETWEEN SIGNS AND SYMPTOMS OF OPIATE WITHDRAWAL AND INITIAL METHADONE DOSE

	Signs and Symptoms	Initial Methadone Dose
Grade 1:	Lacrimation, rhinorrhea, diaphoresis, yawning, restlessness, and insomnia	5 mg
Grade 2:	Dilated pupils, piloerection, muscle twitching, myalgia, arthralgia, and abdominal pain	10 mg
Grade 3:	Tachycardia, hypertension, hyperpnea, fever, anorexia, nausea, and extreme restlessness	15 mg
Grade 4:	Diarrhea, vomiting, dehydration, hyperglycemia, hypotension, and curled-up position	20 mg

Note. From "Guidelines for the Management of Hospitalized Narcotic Addicts" by J. M. Fultz and E. C. Senay, *Annals of Internal Medicine*, 1975, 82, 815–818. Copyright 1975. Reprinted by permission.

tion. Since orally administered methadone usually takes 2-4 hours to have any significant effects (30 minutes to 1 hour after parenteral administration), the clinician must not expect withdrawal symptoms to disappear promptly after its administration. In this circumstance, judicious use of additional short-acting narcotics may be necessary to render the patient symptom-free, which may be necessary in the management of the presenting medical problem.

Once stabilization is achieved, a total of 10-30 mg per day of methadone in divided doses will usually constitute an adequate regimen. It is unusual for a patient to require more than 30 mg per day for stabilization in a hospital setting where the total daily dose is divided and given two or three times daily, provided that the physician has not told the patient what dose he or she is being given.

The addition of a short-acting narcotic to suppress symptoms frequently is preferable to raising the dose of methadone during the initial days of hospitalization. Methadone has a slow onset and a protracted duration of action, which is thought to be due to its conversion to an active metabolite that is slowly metabolized or excreted. Thus, following repetitive doses, effects will be greater after 2-3 days in treatment than they are on the first day.

Discharge plans for the "street addict" differ from those for the methadone enrollee. All drug users should be referred to the hospital's social service department as soon as possible after admission to formulate an outpatient treatment plan or be referred to an appropriate treatment program. Three options are available. The patient can choose to be enrolled in a drug abuse program, be detoxified, or simply be discharged.

Drug dependent patients who want to enroll in a methadone maintenance program must meet the Food and Drug Administration's (FDA) prerequisites. Even when all requirements are satisfied, the reality is that treatment resources for eligible drug dependent persons are severely limited in most areas of the United States. The physician often will have to prepare his patient for a waiting period that may extend into months. The actuality of a long delay may tempt the physician to support the patient's habit. This illegal and dangerous impulse must be resisted. A useful alternative that the physician can offer is detoxification in a hospital setting.

Patients who elect detoxification can usually tolerate a daily reduction of from 5-20% of the total dose without severe discomfort. The dose of methadone can be decreased on a daily basis, or at 2-day intervals, but the intake should always keep withdrawal symptoms at a tolerable level. Supplementary tranquilizers may be necessary in managing such patients.

Finally, it must be recognized that some patients will choose to return to their former lifestyles. Substantial clinical experience suggests that it is a dangerous practice and forbidden by law to prescribe opiates furtively or for nonexistent medical indications. Attempts by individual physicians to treat drug dependence outside of approved treatment programs have been unsuccessful and, in some instances, disastrous.

SURGERY ON THE DRUG AND ALCOHOL ABUSER

The growing incidence of crime, disease, and violence associated with drug abuse has led to surgical problems in the drug dependent person. Unfortunately such patients often do not give reliable histories. The surgeon must exercise a great deal of caution if he or she is to avoid unexpected complications. For example, the drug dependent person's increased tolerance and psychological reliance on narcotics can create a problem for preanesthetic sedation.

Preanesthetic hypotension in drug dependent patients is a problem of which the anesthesiologist and the surgeon must be aware. The use of the naloxone (Narcan) test, when possible, may help to identify the patient who is drug dependent: 0.2-0.4 mg of Narcan is administered intravenously producing pupillary dilation in a patient who has recently received narcotics. Otherwise, pupillary size in these patients can be unreliable in determining anesthetic plans.

An important general principle in managing the drug dependent patient is that surgical trauma should not be accompanied by an attempt to detoxify the patient. The classic case is that of the heroin dependent patient who must undergo surgery for a gunshot or knife wound. The patient should not be caused to undergo the stresses of surgery and withdrawal at the same time. The patient should be maintained on opiates at least until he or she has recovered from surgery; the drug of choice is methadone (Dolophine). The dose of methadone needed to maintain patients in hospitals is relatively low. There are few opiate dependent persons who cannot be maintained in a hospital setting on 10 mg of parenteral methadone administered two or three times daily. This is also true of methadone maintenance patients on high doses of methadone. Although if oral administration is possible, the dose administered prior to hospitalization should be continued in the hospital.

Analgesic needs are not met by the administration of methadone in opiate dependent individuals. Analgesic needs of surgical patients appear to be completely independent of the narcotic habit. Meperidine (Demerol), therefore, should be used in ordinary analgesic doses while the patient is being maintained on methadone. Pentazocine (Talwin) *should not be used* as an analgesic because it can precipitate withdrawal in an opiate dependent individual.

Awareness of preexistent or currently active liver disease is also essential to good anesthetic and surgical practice with the patient who is drug dependent. Postoperatively, the unsuspected drug dependent patient may show signs of congestive heart failure or pulmonary edema with lack of evidence of fluid overload. This relates directly to the pulmonary edema seen in overdose problems and requires careful monitoring and intensive therapy. The surgeon should think of narcotic abuse in any young person, particularly those admitted with stab and gunshot wounds or any injury that might be suspected as one occurring in the world of the drug abuser. This increased awareness might also prevent the occurrence of postoperative withdrawal symptoms occasionally seen in these patients.

Postoperative ileus following abdominal surgery in drug dependent patients has been reported, but its association with drug abuse is not clear-cut. The patient may complain of inordinate amounts of postoperative pain to obtain his "fix" from the unsuspecting surgeon. When this situation persists, interviewing members of the family often will elicit a more accurate history. Occasionally, drug dependent patients will obtain "street stuff" from their friends or family and may behave so as to totally disrupt the hospital environment. The surgeon should not hesitate to use hospital guards and the full range of his authority to respond to such behavior. Psychiatric consultations, if available, should be sought.

An important issue in surgical treatment of the drug dependent patient is what to do about the patient's dependency after surgery. The patient can be detoxified from drugs once the surgical crisis is past, but management of drug dependent patients on general hospital wards is difficult. In most circumstances, the best decision is to discharge the patient to the street with referral to the nearest drug abuse program or specialist. Although this may appear to be an unpalatable solution, there may be few alternatives. The internist or surgeon who tries to dispense opiates to opiate dependent patients usually ends up being manipulated and contributing to illegal distribution of the drug. The surgeon should be aware that most drug dependent persons will sell opiates and/or tranquilizers on the street. Psychoactive drugs have a very substantial "street" value, so there is strong economic incentive to manipulate physicians.

The physician should tell the patient that by law he cannot maintain him or her on opiate drugs. The FDA rules prohibit the average practitioner from dispensing methadone to anyone for more than 21 days. This dispensing limitation is solely for use in a hospital and solely for detoxification. The surgeon should recommend that the patient seek help in a drug abuse program. In such programs the patient can relate more easily to the treatment setting where proper safeguards for diversion may be instituted.

Finally, the surgeon should examine his or her attitude toward the drug dependent person. The attitude of a physician may be directly reflected in the amount of anesthesia, analgesics, sedatives, and tranquilizers required by a patient. An extremely important aspect of responding to the needs of the heroin dependent is the attitude of the staff of the hospital. Most physicians are not trained properly in drug dependence. They are liable to regard the drug dependent person as they have historically regarded the alcoholic, as someone undesirable who does not have the same status as persons with other diseases. Such an attitude may be communicated to hospital staff. If it is, it is not a realistic basis on which to deal with the medical and surgical needs of any human being. Management of the drug dependent patient is frequently difficult, and the physician cannot move from categorical rejection to categorical acceptance. The drug dependent patient's attitude is frequently negative; he or she often may be manipulative and attempt to use the relationship in selfish ways. A more constructive attitude for the surgeon is to try to learn about the drug dependent patient and his or her world while dealing with his or her medical needs. This often requires a great deal of patience and a willingness to understand the patient's lifestyle.

ANALGESIA FOR DRUG DEPENDENT PATIENTS

Methadone maintained patients may require analgesia for other medical problems. These needs can usually be met with normal doses of dihydromorphinone (Dilaudid), meperidine (Demerol), or morphine in addition to the maintenance dose of methadone. The drug dependent person's tolerance to narcotics shortens the time of analgesic effect.

Therefore, most maintenance patients will require more frequent administration of the analgesic than a "naive" patient.

Dihydromorphinone, meperidine, and morphine are safe and effective analgesics. *Pentazocine (Talwin), however, must never be administered to a methadone maintained or heroin dependent patient because this analgesic is also a narcotic antagonist and will precipitate an abstinence syndrome.*

MANAGEMENT OF THE INFANT WITHDRAWAL SYNDROME

Various studies place the frequency of the withdrawal syndrome in neonates of opiate dependent mothers between 40% and 85%.

Treatment for this neonatal condition is usually straightforward: paregoric (4-8 drops), phenobarbital (8-10 mg/kg/day in four divided oral doses), or chlorpromazine (2.8 mg/kg/day in four divided oral doses).

Diazepam has also been effective, but its routine use is not recommended because the parenteral form has sodium benzoate as a preservative. Sodium benzoate inhibits albumin binding of indirect bilirubin, which may enhance the development of bilirubin encephalopathy in jaundiced infants.

ALCOHOLICS IN THE GENERAL HOSPITAL

As noted earlier, the physician should have a high index of suspicion for alcoholism. This is especially true in the general hospital where alcoholism is frequently unrecognized until it is in its end stages.

Careful history-taking for all hospitalized patients coupled with an awareness of community facilities and self-help groups can result in early and successful intervention. There is growing evidence that until it is in its end stages, alcoholism is a highly treatable condition. While a patient is being treated for a concurrent medical or surgical problem, he or she can be linked with AA groups, work with the family can be started, and referrals to community resources can be completed.

Use of alcoholism screening tests may aid in case findings, but the most important variable is the physician's recognition of the frequency of public health problems related to alcohol abuse in our society and our obligation as physicians to find and treat reversible diseases.

REFERENCES

American Psychiatric Association Task Force on Drug Dependence. Position statement on guidelines for methadone maintenance treatment by private psychiatrists. *American Journal of Psychiatry,* 1971, *128,* 254-255.

Fultz, J. M., & Senay, E. C. Guidelines for the management of hospitalized narcotic addicts. *Annals of Internal Medicine,* 1975, *82,* 815-818.

14
Pharmacotherapy of Drug and Alcohol Abusing Patients

GENERAL COMMENTS ON CHEMOTHERAPY, NARCOTIC ADDICTION, AND ALCOHOLISM

Pharmacotherapy now plays a major role in the treatment of heroin addiction and addiction to other opiate drugs. In addition to the widespread use of methadone maintenance for this purpose, a long-acting form of methadone, *l*-alpha-acetylmethadol (LAAM), and a narcotic antagonist, naltrexone, have gained a more limited acceptance in the treatment of opiate addiction. In the treatment of alcoholism, disulfiram (Antabuse) has proved a useful adjunct to the long-term treatment of the alcoholic.

METHADONE MAINTENANCE

Methadone maintenance, pioneered by Dole and Nyswander (1965), is the current treatment of choice for many chronic opiate dependent persons. The consensus of workers in the field is that drug treatment programs using methadone in support of their efforts can be useful for some 40-60% of opiate dependent persons and can aid them to achieve a socially desirable change in lifestyle. Currently there are over 70,000 persons in methadone maintenance programs.

Methadone, a synthetic opiate, is subjectively similar to morphine in that effective analgesia follows the injection of 5-10 mg. In sufficiently high dosage in nontolerant individuals, it has euphorigenic effects comparable to those experienced from the use of heroin. The duration of methadone-induced analgesia is similar to that of heroin (3-4 hours), but withdrawal discomfort in methadone dependent users does not commence for 12-24 hours, while heroin withdrawal occurs after 4-6 hours. The extended "holding" period of methadone plus the fact that methadone is orally effective, defines its usefulness in treating opiate dependency. Orally administered, one dose of methadone during maintenance effectively prevents the appearance of the abstinence syndrome for 24 hours. Heroin, on the other hand, requires frequent parenteral administration.

In the classic work of Dole and Nyswander, methadone maintenance involved an initial period of induction in which the patient was first given oral methadone sufficient to eliminate withdrawal symptoms. Over a period of several weeks this dose was gradually raised to a "blocking" dose of approximately 100 mg/day. Reported side effects were minimal, and opiate "hunger" was eliminated. Not only did this dose eliminate opiate "hunger," but tolerance to opioids was raised to such a degree that normal doses of "street" heroin had no effect, i.e., they were "blocked." It was believed that loss of the positive reinforcement from heroin administration would lead to extinction of the habit.

Dole and Nyswander's original studies limited admissions to male patients 21-39 years old with at least a 5-year history of heroin dependency and a record of previous (nonmethadone) treatment failures. Excluded were psychotics, alcoholics, medically ill, and mentally deficient patients.

Results from these early studies were promising. Approximately two-thirds of the patients were still in treatment after 42 months, and many of the dropouts had subsequently joined other treatment programs. Arrest rates declined, while social adjustment, as measured by return to school and legitimate employment, improved. It was noted that approximately 10% of the patients simply changed drugs of abuse to alcohol, cocaine, barbiturates, or amphetamines, and many of these were expelled, discharged, or terminated from treatment.

On the basis of this and similar experience, methadone maintenance has gained growing acceptance. More recent studies have indicated lower success rates in other programs, an effect no doubt attributable to more open admissions, i.e., accepting psychotics, alcoholics, and other high-risk drug dependent persons into treatment.

Appropriate methadone dosage remains a controversial question. Goldstein and Judson (1973) have demonstrated that program outcome remains equally desirable regardless of doses, i.e., 40-50 mg schedules in comparison to the original 100-120 mg schedule of Dole and Nyswander. Apparently the ability of a high dose to block the effects of heroin is not as important as the relief of opioid craving, which may be effectively achieved at the lower dose. Patients given 15-40 mg daily may initially complain of discomfort beginning 16-18 hours after administration, but they seem to adapt readily to the 24-hour schedule.

Urinalysis for the detection of the use of methadone, heroin, and other drugs has become an integral part of maintenance treatment. Those dependent on opiates are frequently unreliable in reporting drug-related activities, and urinalysis is a convenient technique for obtaining independent data. It may also serve a deterrent purpose, by increasing the likelihood that drug use will be detected. When used as a technique for fostering honesty, urine monitoring can be helpful.

A typical methadone maintenance clinic provides daily administration of oral methadone, plus such "ancillary" services as vocational, legal, and social counseling. Group therapy is normally provided, but this is usually optional. The nature of the groups tends to be confrontational, with an emphasis on honesty and direct reporting of feelings. This approach leads to intense emotional experiences, and some patients find the intensity of the groups so anxiety provoking that they cannot derive benefit from them.

Although the provision of counseling and ancillary social services in methadone treatment has not yet been conclusively proven to influence treatment outcome, few serious observers doubt the vital role that such services play.

Usually, there are subgroups of drug dependent persons who enter most treatment programs. One subgroup may be highly motivated and will improve whether or not actively engaged in treatment. Another group may have such low motivation and be so burdened with social and psychological pathology that no treatment will produce any change. Outcome of a third, intermediate group is probably strongly dependent on the quality of ancillary treatment services.

Ex-opiate dependent individuals are often involved as counselors in drug treatment programs. They are usually highly motivated and uniquely knowledgeable with respect to the meaning of behaviors and experiences of patients from the drug subculture. Some believe that they provide an important role in mediating the sociocultural gap between physicians and patients. They also serve as role models for new patients. The precise role of the ex-drug dependent worker in methadone maintenance clinics remains to be developed fully. Programs vary widely in the extent to which they utilize ex-drug dependent persons, and few meaningful studies have been carried out to help define the role and potential of this important class of workers.

It is unclear whether traditional psychotherapy is useful for most patients on methadone maintenance. Provision of chemical support and the general affiliation with a program seem to be more important, but extensive psychotherapy is clearly indicated among those patients manifesting psychopathology that is amenable to such treatment. The role of anxiolytic and antidepressant agents in methadone maintenance patients is not clear but in some instances such agents can be useful.

Current FDA regulations require detoxification of opiate dependent patients who have been dependent for less than 2 years; detoxification schedules for such patients are prescribed by FDA regulations and cannot extend beyond 21 days. Individuals whose dependence on heroin has lasted longer than 2 years are eligible for methadone maintenance, for which there is no prescribed termination point.

COMMON CLINICAL PROBLEMS IN METHADONE MAINTENANCE PATIENTS

Methadone, as it is used in maintenance programs, has several common side effects, including sedation, constipation, excessive sweating, urinary retention, and changes in sex drive (usually a decrease, but occasionally an increase). Present data indicates that prolonged opiate use of any kind reduces the elaboration of testosterone. The significance of these effects is not clear. Rarely, pruritus, urticaria, and nausea have been reported. Appetite may improve with the consequent development of a weight problem.

Clinical experience in the treatment of heroin dependent patients suggests that the psychophysiological changes attendant upon the person's attempt to change his or her lifestyle are usually more significant than those pharmacologically induced by methadone. Tolerance to most side effects usually develops quickly, except for constipation (which develops early in treatment but usually subsides).

Caution should be exercised in the administration of CNS depressants for anxiety or sedation because of the possibility of synergism with methadone. Benzodiazepines can be given in small doses during critical periods.

Methadone has been used to maintain pregnant women through delivery. Surprisingly, few newborns of such patients exhibit withdrawal syndromes, but such cases, when they arise, may be treated with small doses of paregoric, or if convulsions are a problem, phenobarbital can be used. Possible teratogenic or abortifacient properties of methadone have not yet been conclusively ruled out, but when weighing the risks of maintaining pregnant patients on methadone, one must bear in mind that hazards to the fetus are implicit in the lifestyle of the heroin dependent individual. One must also remember that prematurity is a common occurrence in newborns of the pregnant heroin dependent person but is not a common occurrence in newborns of methadone maintained mothers.

Physicians working in drug abuse programs usually elect to maintain pregnant opiate dependent women on low doses (15-30 mg) of methadone throughout pregnancy and delivery. The use of high-dose methadone appears to be associated with the same perinatal morbidity and mortality as use of "street" heroin. Withdrawal in pregnant women, particularly in the third trimester, is thought to be dangerous to the fetus. Not using methadone at all is equivalent to returning the patient to the street where she usually continues to use narcotics as well as a variety of other drugs.

The most common serious complication in patients on methadone maintenance therapy is alcoholism. O'Donnell (1969) reports that two-thirds of the drug dependent persons seen at Lexington have a history of alcohol excess, so it is not surprising that when opiate dependency is controlled by methadone therapy, cases of alcohol abuse appear. A patient showing signs of acute alcohol intoxication should not receive methadone while he or she is intoxicated. Alcohol and methadone are synergistic, and a lethal outcome is possible. A methadone program should offer special programming for the alcoholic drug dependent person whenever possible. This may involve the creation of a special unit that offers alcohol detoxification, disulfiram therapy, and/or referral to Alcoholics Anonymous (AA).

Methadone maintenance, i.e., a treatment contract in which the patient expects to receive methadone daily for the indefinite future, is indicated for heroin dependent persons who are not strongly motivated to achieve immediate abstinence. Methadone maintenance therapy does not have the goal of "complete cure," if by this phrase we mean complete and permanent abstention from all opiate drugs and full social rehabilitation. Goals of methadone maintenance are, at a minimum, reduction of illicit drug use, reduction of criminal activity, increase in productivity as reflected by employment in the legitimate job market, and increase in self-esteem. In addition, improvement in family and community functioning is sought.

Some have attacked the basic premise of methadone maintenance, maintaining that methadone is an opiate and as such does not cure opiate dependency and that abstinence is the only meaningful criterion of cure. With increasing experience, however, it has become clear that a significant percentage of opiate dependent individuals will not become abstinent under the various treatment methods now known. In the light of this observation, it appears that methadone maintenance can provide help to a large number of persons who would otherwise be returned to full-scale criminal activity and illicit drug use. It must be borne in mind that the typical opiate dependent person normally uses illegal heroin that is both expensive and impure. While the drug addict faces arrest for using heroin, maintaining the habit becomes a full-time job. On the other hand, medically sponsored methadone administration is legal and safe. It permits the opiate dependent person to seek employment, choose friends more freely, and lead a more stable life. Psychologically, the status associated with chronic heroin dependency is destructive to self-esteem. By being "on methadone," a patient can feel that he or she is taking medicine instead of "drugs," and can start to feel some socially sanctioned basis for self-esteem. The treatment clinic can provide support and treatment for primary or secondary psychosocial problems. With community-based control of clinics, the argument that methadone maintenance is used as a social control mechanism does not appear to be compelling.

It is too soon to make any definitive statements regarding the future role of methadone maintenance. At present, it appears that methadone maintenance has an important role in the development of a national treatment strategy for problems of drug dependence. It seems indisputable that a large number of people are now being helped in methadone programs. The evidence also suggests that for the average opiate dependent individual, treatment in a program is preferable to treatment by an individual therapist.

OTHER OPIATE MAINTENANCE

LAAM differs from methadone in that it suppresses the abstinence syndrome for 2-3 days, while methadone suppresses the abstinence syndrome for approximately 24 hours. Experience to date suggests that LAAM is therapeutically quite similar to methadone. In comparison with methadone, LAAM maintenance treatment appears to have the advantages of more flexibility in the way it is dispensed.

Because LAAM only has to be administered three times per week, all of the drug can be administered at the clinic site, thereby minimizing any possibility of illicit diversion. LAAM has been tested thus far on several thousand addicts. For a number of reasons, not the least of which is that LAAM has fewer subjective effects than methadone, methadone is still the preferred maintenance drug among clients; LAAM is unlikely to replace it on a wide scale. For example, the client on methadone, while not experiencing a high, feels the effects of having taken a drug. This feeling is less pronounced wih LAAM. Its voluntary use will probably be limited to the select group of patients who prefer the absence of a subjective drug effect, yet need a drug lasting 2-3 days, or programs that institute its use as a public health measure to eliminate the problems of diversion with "take-home" methadone. At present LAAM is an investigational drug, and not approved for general use.

OTHER OPIOID SUBSTITUTES

For many years scientists have attempted to develop an opioid with effective pain-killing properties but with minimal dependency liability. In the problem of chemotherapy for opiate dependency, this goal becomes one of finding a drug that effectively alleviates opioid craving without significant dependency potential. Recent work with propoxyphene napsylate (Darvon-N) suggests that this drug (chemically similar to methadone) may provide effective relief for opioid craving while having a low dependency potential.

Gay, Senay, and Newmeyer (1973) in one study, and Tennant (1974) in another, have utilized Darvon-N successfully in the detoxification of heroin dependent persons. Tennant et al. also report successful use of Darvon-N in the withdrawal of methadone maintenance patients. Initial doses of Darvon-N are in the 200-400 mg range. The single oral daily dose is then increased if patients request an increase or if clinical conditions dictate. Usual maintenance doses range from 400-1600 mg. A problem in Darvon-N therapy is the relatively narrow range between therapeutic and toxic doses. "Seizure-like" attacks at doses of 100 mg per day have been described by Tennant. Nausea and vomiting, "shakiness," and "spaced out" feelings are described in patients studied by Gay et al. Darvon-N therapy at this time constitutes a controversial area of research. This drug is not approved for general use at present.

In this context it should be noted that animal experiments with many hundreds of opioids suggest that if one ranks such drugs in terms of pain-killing effectiveness, exactly the same ranking applies to their respective ability to relieve abstinence and also to their dependency potential. If propoxyphene napsylate or some other drug proves not to follow this rule, the implications are of course highly significant for treatment. Darvon-N is an investigational drug at this time.

NARCOTIC ANTAGONISTS

There are drugs such as naloxone, cyclazocine, and naltrexone that directly antagonize opiate effects in the human body. Recently, much work has been devoted to their possible utility in the treatment of opiate dependency. This technique is roughly analogous to the use of disulfiram in the treatment of alcoholism except that disulfiram creates a situation in which the use of alcohol precipitates negative effects, while narcotic antagonists simply block the effects of opiates.

The most promising narcotic antagonist for the treatment of opiate addiction is naltrexone, a modification of the naloxone molecule. Like naloxone, it is essentially a pure antagonist with virtually no agonist (morphine-like) effects. Yet, unlike naloxone, it has a long duration of action. Therefore, naltrexone is a drug that while itself is not addicting, can completely block the effects of injected heroin.

Naltrexone can be taken orally on a daily or a triweekly basis. Unlike an earlier antagonist drug, cyclazocine, naltrexone has virtually no unpleasant side effects. Its safety and effectiveness are now undergoing clinical investigation; approximately 5,000 addicts have been treated with it. Thus far it appears that naltrexone is a safe and effective drug. Candidates for antagonist treatment must be completely opiate-free, since antagonists induce severe and conceivably lethal withdrawal syndromes if administered to opiate dependent patients.

While the average heroin dependent person who takes naltrexone does so for relatively short periods (a few weeks), a few stay on the drug for as long as a year. However, only a small number of heroin addicts have volunteered to take it, and for this reason it may have a relatively small impact on the total treatment effort. Preliminary studies of the drug's effectiveness show that it has provided significant support for heroin abstinence and is positively correlated with the achievement of social rehabilitative goals. Whether the positive results are due to the antagonist drug itself or are simply an indication that the group electing to take it is more highly motivated, naltrexone (Trexan) is likely to remain an important but limited adjunct to treatment during the transition from detoxification to continued abstinence.

ANTABUSE (DISULFIRAM)

No drug by itself should be considered *the* treatment for alcoholism. However, drugs can play the role as an adjunct to such treatment.

Alcohol is broken down in the liver into acetaldehyde, which is then converted to carbon dioxide and water. Antabuse (disulfiram) blocks the enzyme, aldehyde dehydrogenase, which mediates this reaction. Thus, Antabuse interferes with the breakdown of acetaldehyde, causing elevations of acetaldehyde in the blood sufficient to produce nausea, flushing, dysphoria, dyspnea, hypertension, and syncope. Heart failure and in rare instances death is possible. Antabuse is used by many clinicians, but its efficacy has not been established on a scientific basis.

Patients starting Antabuse therapy need to be free of alcohol for 12 hours. The dose and frequency of administration varies from clinician to clinician, but the usual procedure is to give a 500 mg loading dose for 5 days followed by a daily maintenance dose of 250 mg. Some clinicians prescribe it three times a week, but most prescribe it for daily use. If patients taking Antabuse drink any alcohol whatsoever, they are apt to have a reaction. Even the alcohol in aftershave lotion absorbed through the skin can cause a reaction in very sensitive people. Nonetheless, a thorough indoctrination concerning the many foods and products containing alcohol is required before starting this drug. From practical experience, the most common inadvertent ingestion of alcohol occurs with medications in elixir form. Usually, alcoholics taking disulfiram who cannot maintain sobriety will stop the drug for a few days before they resume drinking. Most who resume drinking after stopping Antabuse for 7-10 days will experience no adverse reaction. To be on the safe side, patients are advised to wait for at least 14 days. If they drink while taking Antabuse, they will have a reaction which is dependent on both the dose of Antabuse and alcohol. This Antabuse-alcohol reaction can constitute a serious medical emergency. The treatment of such reactions is symptomatic, e.g., treatment of shock by ordinary measures. Inhalation of 95% oxygen and 5% carbon dioxide is thought to be useful by some clinicians. Ascorbic acid has also been used.

Use of Antabuse in severe end-stage alcoholics can be dangerous and if the clinician has evidence that the alcoholic is unable to stop use of alcohol, he or she should attempt to control the situation by means other than Antabuse.

Antabuse should be used with caution in patients with major medical problems such as diabetes, cerebral damage, epilepsy, and renal problems, and is contraindicated in patients who are allergic to the drug, psychotic, or who have severe coronary artery disease. Antabuse itself, in some individuals, may cause mild sedation, confusion, and carbon disulfide poisoning. The clinician should monitor the patient taking Antabuse for neurological problems secondary to carbon disulfide poisoning. Carbon disulfide is one of the major metabolites of disulfiram. There are a few cases in which Antabuse is thought to have caused hepatotoxicity. Antabuse also potentiates the effects of certain drugs, for example, phenytoin coumarin derivatives and isoniazid, and is relatively contraindicated when these drugs are used. It is not an innocuous drug, and its chronic use should be carefully monitored. Antabuse should only be prescribed with the patient's full knowledge and consent.

For many patients Antabuse provides insurance against the impulse to drink and can free up energy for other pursuits. It is compatible with other forms of alcoholism treatment and is particularly useful with the difficult to treat binge-drinking alcoholics.

While many thousands of alcoholics have been helped by taking Antabuse, those who do best are those with the best prognosis initially. The degree of its effectiveness, therefore, is still a matter of some scientific debate. Nonetheless, many physicians feel that Antabuse is a unique and important contribution to the recovery of their alcoholic patients.

OTHER DRUGS

Tranquilizers, particularly the benzodiazepines Librium and Valium, have been used to treat the anxiety symptoms of recovering sober alcoholics or as an adjunct to efforts assisting the individual to regain some moderate drinking behavior. Clinical experience with these drugs as a "substitute" for alcohol has been disappointing. More often than not alcohol is used excessively along with these drugs, increasing the risk of intoxication and lethal overdose. Experience with addiction shows that once control is lost with alcohol, it is often lost with other sedative-hypnotics. Only in very exceptional situations is their use recommended as a substitute for alcohol or as an adjunct to alcoholism treatment.

Tricyclic antidepressants and lithium have a specialized and sometimes beneficial effect on the sober recovering alcoholic who has depressive or manic symptoms. Caution should be exercised with tricyclics because if the patient continues to drink excessively, the combination of alcohol and tricyclics greatly enhances the risk of harmful overdose reactions.

REFERENCES

Dole, V. P., & Nyswander, M. A medical treatment for diacetylmorphine (heroin) addiction: A clinical trial with methadone hydrochloride. *Journal of the American Medical Association,* 1965, *193,* 646-650.

Gay, G. R., Senay, E. C., & Newmeyer, J. A. The pseudo junkie: Evolution of heroin life style in the non-addicted individual. *Drug Forum,* 1973, *2,* 279-290.

Goldstein, A., & Judson, B. A. Efficacy and side effects of three widely different methadone doses. In *Proceedings of the Fifth National Conference on Methadone Treatment.* New York: National Association for the Prevention of Addiction to Narcotics, 1973.

O'Donnell, J. A. *Narcotic addicts in Kentucky* (U.S. Public Health Service Publication No. 1881). Washington, D.C.: U.S. Government Printing Office, 1969.

Tennant, F. S., Jr. Propoxyphene napsylate (Darvon-N) treatment of heroin addicts. *Journal of the National Medical Association,* 1974, *66,* 23-24, 27.

15
Sociotherapy of Drug and Alcohol Abusers

The term "sociotherapy" denotes many different approaches to the treatment of drug abuse. Their underlying common element is that they put primary emphasis on social interaction. Some forbid all "chemicals" as a matter of policy, while others may use drugs quite extensively. However, chemotherapy is at most an adjunct to treatment and does not itself constitute treatment.

THERAPEUTIC COMMUNITIES

The "therapeutic community" technique of drug abuse rehabilitation (not to be confused with the phrase coined to describe the milieu therapy of Maxwell Jones in psychiatric wards) was created by Charles Diederich in the late 1950's. Diederich, a "graduate" of Alcoholics Anonymous, began holding meetings for alcoholics. Several drug abusers started coming to these meetings, and Diederich became interested in their problems. By the early 1960's the structure of Synanon, Diederich's notion of drug rehabilitation and the archetypal therapeutic community, was completely developed. Since then, therapeutic communities have flourished throughout the country.

Diederich's basic concept is that a person who uses drugs is emotionally immature and, as a consequence, cannot function in "straight" society. Treatment in the typical therapeutic community lasts 1-2 years, after which the person will reenter the "outside" community as a successfully functioning, drug-free individual. During this treatment period, psychological growth, measured in phases or steps in the various programs, proceeds until a client has acquired the ability to function autonomously.

In general, therapeutic communities are based on the notion that an individual knows his or her feelings and can report them if he or she desires to do so. There is an emphasis on honesty and a directness of approach that is unquestionably therapeutic for many. Typically, intake requires considerable initiative on the part of the prospective resident. During what is usually a stressful "intake interview," the candidate must actively and vigorously commit himself or herself to the program. Such a situation serves the double purpose of screening out candidates of low motivation (for whom therapeutic communities are probably inappropriate) and providing a very explicit and self-defined reason for the successful candidate to enter treatment. Upon admission, social status is low. The new resident has no "privileges," i.e., there are restrictions on telephone calls, personal possessions, visitors, and the like. Typically, the neophyte is given rather poor living quarters, is assigned menial tasks, and is expected to follow all house rules (e.g., no drugs, physical violence, or disobeying orders). The resident is expected to function well in his or her job, to manifest concern about fellow residents, and to be active in group therapy sessions. If these expectations are met, the resident will progress through successful phases in which autonomy is given incrementally.

A well-functioning therapeutic community could be compared to a very large and tightly run family. Indeed the word "family" is often used to denote the entire membership of a therapeutic community. Punishment for inappropriate behavior in the form of verbal "haircuts," demeaning tasks, and peer contempt can be quite severe in some therapeutic communities. In this respect the form of treatment provided by therapeutic communities may not be beneficial for younger patients or adolescents who are plagued by low self-esteem and weak ego structure.

Encounter groups, led by staff and/or advanced residents, are held frequently. Usually, a resident will participate in three such groups each week. Honesty of expression and open verbal hostility are considered proper group behavior. Such groups are helpful in resolving personal problems in a psychotherapeutic sense and in providing an appropriate setting for "blowing off steam" for people living under stressful conditions.

Reentry into the community outside is usually divided into several steps. The patient progresses from being a regular resident with some personal freedom, e.g., weekend passes, visitors, etc., to living outside the therapeutic community while attending occasional therapeutic community groups. After considerable time in a basically outpatient status, the ex-drug dependent patient formally graduates from the therapeutic community (assuming no relapse) and is formally considered rehabilitated.

In visiting a therapeutic community, one is struck by the high esprit de corps of the family, the personal friendliness of the residents, and the sense of order apparent in the cleanliness of the house. Certain aspects of the community, such as the extreme control of the individual and the intolerance of minor deviance, may be disquieting. A new resident is traditionally expected to detoxify from heroin "cold turkey," i.e., without any chemical support. During withdrawal, he or she is expected to participate fully in house activities. One finds that subjective withdrawal symptoms under such circumstances, where passivity is not permitted, are far less unpleasant than when "kicking" in a hospital or jail.

The most serious problem in the therapeutic community approach is a very high premature termination of treatment or "split" rate. Although accurate statistics are difficult to compile, it is estimated that slightly less than 10% of new members will ever graduate. The majority of splits occur in the first few months of treatment, but splitting at a lower rate continues up to graduation.

Observers have noted that residents who have stayed even a few months before splitting can derive benefit from their stay. Therapeutic communities probably provide the highest quality of rehabilitation of any major treatment modality in that their graduates are drug-free, have a low recidivism rate, and are gifted workers with the drug dependent. A high proportion of graduates get jobs as ex-addict counselors in drug abuse programs. This continued involvement in the rehabilitation process may well account for the low recidivism rate among the graduates who work in such positions. However, therapeutic communities have a tendency to produce graduates who are more fitted to this particular form of employment than to any other. In this respect, therapeutic communities tend to lack breadth in their rehabilitation goals.

The therapeutic community may be the treatment of choice for the very highly motivated drug abuser who has been deeply involved with drugs. It may be dangerous as a form of treatment for some who are unable to identify and/or to report their feelings. The milieu is not generally supportive to people who are unable to function well, although there are some striking exceptions in which psychotics with much previous ineffective traditional treatment have made major recoveries. Although the cost of treatment in this modality is higher than that of methadone maintenance, it has a much greater ability to make significant, long-lasting changes in the lifestyle of the drug abuser. Moreover, it can provide treatment to individuals for whom methadone support is inappropriate, such as polydrug users. However, work in San Francisco (Wesson, Smith, & Lerner, 1975) and Boston (Raynes, Patch, & Cohen, 1975) has shown that, in general, polydrug abusers tend to be more psychiatrically disturbed than pure heroin users. Furthermore, many therapeutic communities tend to find polydrug abusers too disruptive to integrate into their programs.

Although therapeutic communities traditionally have avoided interaction with professionals, this has changed in recent years. At this point, professionals can make significant contributions to therapeutic communities by acting as general consultants. They may also train staff or provide treatment for residents with significant psychiatric problems. Physicians who work with therapeutic communities will do well if they regard themselves as students of the therapeutic-community process and are identified as such by the residents.

MODIFIED THERAPEUTIC COMMUNITIES

There have been many efforts to modify therapeutic communities to permit other subgroups of drug abusers to benefit from the therapeutic-community experience. Jaffe, Zaks, and Washington (1969) developed the multimodality treatment system in which methadone support is incorporated into the therapeutic-community structure. Due to early polarization between drug-free and drug-supported treatment, it was first thought that such a combination would not be feasible. Jaffe's experience, however, has shown that abstinent and methadone-supported patients can be successfully treated in the same unit both on an outpatient and a residential basis. Such "mixed" treatment provides significant programmatic flexibility and the ability to tailor treatment to the specific needs of the individual patient. It is too early to make conclusions regarding comparative outcome measures, but clinical impressions suggest that programs offering "mixed" treatment may reach many who would not succeed in outpatient methadone maintenance or in a traditional therapeutic community.

In the modified therapeutic community, one can observe considerable loosening of the rigid structure of the classic therapeutic community. The loosening takes many forms, from shortening the length of residence (in modified therapeutic communities, length of stay may be in terms of weeks) to reducing stressful aspects of treatment and to increasing the personal freedom of residents. Early results indicate that such modifications may render therapeutic communities less suitable for the groups originally helped by them, but more suitable for other groups, particularly young polydrug users.

OTHER SOCIOTHERAPIES

Sociotherapeutic approaches also include the various religion-oriented drug rehabilitation programs, such as Teen Challenge (a fundamentalist Christian program), the Black Muslims (who base their work on the teachings of Elijah Mohammed), and several small sects using various Eastern philosophies. Many such organizations provide significant help to substantial groups of drug abusers. There are also programs that, while not based on religion, center their efforts on the charisma of a single person. Probably much of their success stems from the same process that enables therapeutic communities to provide structure, affiliation, and hope for their members.

There have been several types of treatment designed specifically for young polydrug abusers. Examples of such alternative treatment agencies are hotlines, drop-in centers, and free clinics. Hotlines are telephone services offering crisis intervention and various types of other services, with the exception of primary care. These services, which began to appear in large numbers in the late 1960's, were set up originally to handle "bad trips." They are typically staffed by young volunteers. Professional supervision of such efforts is desirable, as these programs probably suffered in the past from lack of professional interest. Nonetheless, these services have been meaningful for many young people, and their integration into a network of services would magnify the real contribution they have made.

Drop-in centers may also provide crisis intervention, but they are usually medium-term centers. Many people, particularly the young, will not seek formal treatment, as they are reluctant to consider themselves "sick." Drop-in centers provide an acceptable alternative for treatment. The typical center avoids all medical jargon. An attempt is made to provide recreation and friends, "rap groups," and individual conversations with staff.

It is noteworthy that both drop-in centers and hotlines tend to be operated by very young people with few ties to the medical "establishment," and who often will not trust medical personnel to help them.

Free clinics, of which there are currently over 500 nationwide, provide direct medical, dental, psychological, and drug rehabilitation services. Additionally, they are an important source of credible drug information for the young user who feels that "establishment drug education" is essentially dishonest. The staffs of free clinics are generally composed of volunteer doctors, nurses, lab technicians, counselors, and other trained paraprofessional and nonprofessional personnel.

AA, AL-ANON, AND ALATEEN

Alcoholics Anonymous (AA) was founded in 1935 by a surgeon and a businessman. Since its inception, it probably has helped many millions of people and has given every indication that it will continue to be the most potent of all sources of help for alcoholics. AA is a unique organization—it has no organizational hierarchy; it has no officers; it owns no property; it espouses no political doctrine. Its basic beliefs are embodied in its famous "twelve steps":

1. We admitted we were powerless over alcohol—that our lives have become unmanageable.
2. Came to believe that a power greater than ourselves could restore us to sanity.
3. Made a decision to turn our will and our lives over to the care of God as we understood Him.
4. Made a searching and fearless moral inventory of ourselves.
5. Admitted to God, ourselves, and to another human being the exact nature of our wrongs.
6. We are entirely ready to have God remove all these defects of character.
7. Humbly, we ask Him to remove our shortcomings.
8. Made a list of all persons we had harmed, and became willing to make amends to them all.
9. Made direct amends to such people wherever possible, except when to do so would injure them or others.
10. Continued to take personal inventory, and when we were wrong, promptly admitted it.

11. Sought through prayer and meditation to improve our conscious contact with God as we understood Him, praying only for knowledge of His will for us and the power to carry that out.
12. Having had a spiritual awakening as the result of these steps, we tried to carry this message to alcoholics, and to practice these principles in all our affairs.

AA groups provide hope, a social network free of the ordinary social pressures to drink, a credo, and a crisis response system that is around-the-clock and present wherever the alcoholic might travel. Some specialized AA groups, such as the international AA group for physicians, has many hundreds of members and many local branches which constitute important resources for impaired physicians and their families.

Al-Anon and Alateen were created to assist family members of alcoholics to help themselves and their alcoholic parent, spouse, or relative in whatever way possible. They may be important resources for the physician who elects to work with alcohol abusers.

Philosophically, AA views alcoholism as a disease and is committed to abstinence as the only realistic goal of treatment. Some alcoholics will reject the AA approach because they are unable to put aside the defense of denial, but good management may involve repeated discussion of the potential in AA for the alcoholic.

Attending AA regularly can be a part of every treatment regimen. Attendance appears to provide the emotional support necessary for some alcoholics to resist the strong internal and external pressures to drink. AA teaches that people should conceptualize the struggle as "one day at a time."

COERCIVE TREATMENT

Heroin dependency is uniquely tied to criminality and hence to the criminal justice system. There is no psychopharmacological basis for this association; it occurs principally because the street cost of heroin is high and criminal activity is the only source of funds for the average heroin dependent person.

As a consequence of the social concern over heroin dependency, there are many approaches to involuntary or semivoluntary treatment in lieu of prosecution to civil commitment for drug-related crimes. Results of such approaches to date are inconclusive. The addiction treatment center at Lexington, Kentucky, which had used civil commitment extensively, was criticized by many practitioners, but Vaillant (1973), in a number of long-term follow-up studies, reported rehabilitation rates of about 40%. Wieland and Novack (1973) reported some success in the Philadelphia Criminal Justice Program in which drug dependent persons were offered treatment in lieu of prosecution. However, treatment outcome appears to be poorer than in a comparison group of patients without active relationship to the criminal justice system.

There are many unresolved questions in such approaches regarding treatment efficacy, medical ethics, civil liberties, and social policy. The National Conference of Commissioners on Uniform State Laws (Turner, 1973) proposed guidelines for involuntary treatment, including the following main points:

1. No *mandatory* treatment should be provided except for those who have committed a criminal violation.
2. Mandatory treatment should not be imposed for a longer period than the maximum sentence for the criminal violation, or 18 months, whichever is shorter.
3. The patient should at all times have the option to leave treatment and serve out his or her jail term.
4. The patient should always have the option of drug-free treatment.

Nonvoluntary treatment may become a major tool in drug abuse rehabilitation, but experience to date indicates that where treatment opportunities exist, large numbers of drug dependent individuals will voluntarily seek treatment.

REFERENCES

Jaffe, J. H., Zaks, M. S., & Washington, E. N. Experience with the use of methadone in a multi-modality program for the treatment of narcotics users. *International Journal of the Addictions,* 1969, *4,* 481-490.

Raynes, A. E., Patch, V. D., & Cohen, M. Comparison of opiate and polydrug abusers in treatment. *Journal of Psychedelic Drugs,* 1975, *7,* 135-141.

Turner, L. B. (Ed.) *National Conference of Commissioners on Uniform State Laws: Handbook and proceedings*. Chicago: National Conference of Commissioners on Uniform State Laws. 1973.

Vaillant, G. E. A 20-year follow-up study of New York narcotic addicts. *Archives of General Psychiatry,* 1973, *29,* 237-241.

Wesson, D. R., Smith, D. E., & Lerner, S. E. Streetwise and nonstreetwise polydrug typology: Myth or reality. *Journal of Psychedelic Drugs,* 1975, *7,* 121-124.

Wieland, W. F., & Novack, J. L. A comparison of criminal justice and non-criminal justice related patients in a methadone treatment program. In *Proceedings of the Fifth National Conference on Methadone Treatment*. New York: National Association for the Prevention of Addiction to Narcotics, 1973.

16
Experimental Treatment Modalities

The efforts put forth during the past several years to find effective treatment for those suffering from various forms of drug dependency have taken many and varied directions. Some of those efforts have produced more substantial and more widely accepted results than others. With still other efforts, the experimentation continues. It is this latter category that must be commented upon here.

In each instance, the technique mentioned must be regarded, at present, as a research area. Various claims and counterclaims have been made. All the evidence, however, is not yet in. Time and additional research will provide further insights and perhaps some further answers for the treatment of the drug abusing and/or drug dependent person.

TRANSCENDENTAL MEDITATION

Transcendental meditation has been offered to drug dependent persons throughout the country. The alien aura of this technique to inner-city minority groups plus the requirement that the dependent person must be drug-free for 3 weeks prior to the start of training appear to have prevented meditation from winning wide acceptance with the opiate dependent population. The technique itself appears to be most useful in drug prevention efforts with younger populations who are experimenting with drugs but have not become dependent upon them. Wallace (1970) reports success with such populations in substituting the positive behavior of meditation for the potentially destructive behavior involved with polydrug abuse.

BIOFEEDBACK AND RELAXATION TECHNIQUES

Biofeedback has not been studied on any significant scale in drug dependent populations. It is quite possible that it may have valuable applications. At present, however, much research remains to be carried out. Similar remarks apply to relaxation techniques.

ACUPUNCTURE AND BEHAVIOR MODIFICATION

Both acupuncture and behavior modification (O'Brien, Raynes, & Patch, 1972) have been explored clinically, but there are no published reports of research carried out in a controlled fashion. Thus, evaluation of these techniques is not possible at this time. There would appear to be little question, however, that data will be generated in the near future.

CLONIDINE IN OPIATE WITHDRAWAL

Clonidine hydrochloride, a nonnarcotic antihypertensive, is being investigated because single-dose studies indicate that .005 mg/kg of clonidine gives substantial relief from the opiate withdrawal syndrome. A few studies have been completed and more are under way to determine optimal doses, frequency of doses, safety, and utility both in inpatient and outpatient settings.

Clonidine has been used in treating narcotic dependent persons abruptly ceasing their narcotic intake—for 12-24 hours, .005 mg/kg of clonidine is administered two to three times a day. Over the next 10 days, the dose is titrated on a two- to three-times-a-day schedule according to clinical need. Then, over a 3-day period, the clonidine is phased out with a usual decrement on the 11th day of 50% of the dose on Day 10. The weaning period is necessary because of a possible return of opiate-withdrawal symptoms if clonidine is abruptly stopped. Hypotension, dry mouth, and sedation, sometimes severe, are possible side effects of this regimen. These side effects are treated by decreases in the amount of clonidine and/or frequency of clonidine administration.

Use of clonidine while concurrently withdrawing addicts on decreasing doses of narcotics such as methadone does not appear to intensify each other's sedative effects. The drug appears promising and is being investigated intensively. Clonidine is an experimental drug and is not approved for general use.

REFERENCES

O'Brien, J. S., Raynes, A. E., & Patch, V. D. Treatment of heroin addiction with aversion therapy, relaxation training and systematic desensitization. *Behavior Research and Therapy,* 1972, *10,* 77-80.

Wallace, R. K. Physiological effects of transcendental meditation. *Science,* 1970, *167,* 1751-1754.

17
Treatment Posttest

Answers to the Posttest appear on page 188.

PART I. MULTIPLE CHOICE QUESTIONS
DIRECTIONS: Each item below has five responses. Pick the **one** response that best answers or completes the question and mark the appropriate letter on the answer sheet.

1. Hyperventilation on the part of the drug abusing patient may be a manifestation of—

   ____ A. Acute anxiety.
   ____ B. Metabolic acidosis.
   ____ C. Salicylate poisoning.
   ____ D. Septicemia.
   ____ E. All of the above.

2. A lack of perfusion of vital tissues in the drug abusing patient is diagnosed as shock. This may be caused by—

   ____ A. Fluid loss.
   ____ B. Vasodilation.
   ____ C. Acute allergic reaction.
   ____ D. Systemic infection.
   ____ E. All of the above.

3. The **immediate** objective with the drug abusing patient in the emergency room is to—

   ____ A. Assess and stabilize cardiopulmonary function.
   ____ B. Decrease the absorption of any drug taken orally.

____ C. Administer an appropriate antidote.
____ D. Assess and treat for any evidence of trauma.
____ E. Determine pupillary condition.

4. Drug abusers often present in a comatose state. Which of the following substances of abuse may produce a *cyclic* coma?

____ A. Meprobamate.
____ B. Glutethimide.
____ C. Phencyclidine.
____ D. Cocaine.
____ E. Methaqualone.

5. In using naloxone in the treatment of opiate-overdosed patients, one should remember that—

____ A. The response to administration of antagonists is dramatic and diagnostic.
____ B. It should not be used if a previously conscious patient becomes somnolent.
____ C. It is effective in pentazocine overdose.
____ D. Both B and C.
____ E. Both A and C.

6. Chemotherapeutic management of opiate withdrawal should be accomplished by—

____ A. Administering methadone in constant decrements after the second day.
____ B. Administering chlordiazepoxide in concert with naloxone.
____ C. Administering methadone and beginning decremental reduction when patient is stabilized.
____ D. Administering sedatives with 2-5 mg decrements weekly.
____ E. Administering antipsychotic medication.

7. Certain drugs administered to a person who has recently received narcotics will produce pupillary changes. To determine the presence of narcotics, the appropriate measure is to—

____ A. Administer Nalline (0.2-0.4 mg) orally and look for pupillary constriction.

_____ B. Administer Narcan (0.2-0.4 mg) I.V. and look for pupillary dilation.
_____ C. Administer Narcan (1 mg) orally and look for pupillary constriction.
_____ D. Administer Lorfan (1 mg) and look for pupillary constriction.
_____ E. Administer Nalline (0.2-0.4 mg) orally and look for pupillary dilation.

8. After the last dose of heroin, the longest time that urine screening for morphine can be expected to remain positive is—

_____ A. From 3-6 hours.
_____ B. From 6-12 hours.
_____ C. From 12-24 hours.
_____ D. From 24-72 hours.
_____ E. None of the above.

9. The presence of gross ataxia, nystagmus, and absence of mydriasis are indicative of—

_____ A. Stimulant withdrawal.
_____ B. Opiate intoxication.
_____ C. PCP intoxication.
_____ D. Alcohol withdrawal.
_____ E. Stimulant overdose.

10. The length of time for withdrawal from diazepam to occur following cessation of intake is—

_____ A. 1 day.
_____ B. 2-3 days.
_____ C. 7-10 days.
_____ D. 3 weeks.
_____ E. None of the above.

11. From the appearance of morphine in the urine specimen, it can be concluded that—

_____ A. An opiate has been used within the past 24 hours.
_____ B. The subject is a drug abuser.
_____ C. The subject is a polydrug abuser, if indications of quinine are also found.

182 / The Diagnosis and Treatment of Drug and Alcohol Abuse

    ____ D. The subject is on methadone maintenance.
    ____ E. None of the above can be unequivocably concluded.

12. The most serious problem in the therapeutic community approach is—

    ____ A. A high recidivism rate.
    ____ B. A high "split" rate.
    ____ C. Suicide.
    ____ D. Criminal behavior.
    ____ E. None of the above.

PART II. COMPARISON QUESTIONS

DIRECTIONS: On the answer sheet, make the appropriate answer:

    A, if the item is associated with (A) only
    B, if the item is associated with (B) only
    C, if the item is associated with both (A) and (B)
    D, if the item is associated with neither (A) nor (B)

Questions 13-18

    (A) Diazepam
    (B) Phenytoin
    (C) Both
    (D) Neither

____ 13. Should be administered slowly since cardiac arrest may occur.

____ 14. Long-acting medication not routinely administered in emergency treatment of convulsions.

____ 15. After administration, physician must be alert for cardiopulmonary arrest.

____ 16. Useful as a general anesthesia in seizure treatment.

____ 17. A good antiseizure agent with little sedative properties.

_____ 18. Intramuscular administration is not appropriate because of poor and irregular absorption.

Questions 19-22

  (A) Naloxone
  (B) Thiamine
  (C) Both
  (D) Neither

_____ 19. Normal dosage: 100 mg I.M.

_____ 20. Rapidly reverses all of the depressive effects of narcotics.

_____ 21. Important emergency procedure for the unconscious patient.

_____ 22. Should be given for alcohol overdose.

Questions 23-27

  (A) Stimulants
  (B) Hallucinogens
  (C) Both
  (D) Neither

_____ 23. Nausea.

_____ 24. Hypertension.

_____ 25. Anorexia.

_____ 26. Hypothermia.

_____ 27. Dilated pupils.

PART III. MATCHING QUESTIONS

DIRECTIONS: A patient who has taken a large quantity of CNS depressants is brought to the emergency room in a comatose state. Some of the following measures should be taken routinely, others only under

184 / The Diagnosis and Treatment of Drug and Alcohol Abuse

certain conditions (i.e., if indicated), and others would be inappropriate. Select the one lettered heading that best applies and mark the appropriate letter on the answer sheet.

(A) Routinely
(B) Only if indicated
(C) Not appropriate

28. Perform gastric lavage.

____ A   ____ B   ____ C

29. Provide respiratory support-intubation and mechanical ventilation.

____ A   ____ B   ____ C

30. Continuous monitoring of vital functions.

____ A   ____ B   ____ C

31. Treat with I.V. fluids and a vasopressor.

____ A   ____ B   ____ C

32. Monitor electrolyte balance.

____ A   ____ B   ____ C

33. Administer analeptic drugs.

____ A   ____ B   ____ C

34. Stimulate diuresis.

____ A   ____ B   ____ C

35. Administer analgesics.

____ A   ____ B   ____ C

PART IV. MULTIPLE TRUE AND FALSE
DIRECTIONS: Each of the following items has four choices, one of which may be correct, two of which may be correct, three of which may be correct, or all of which may be correct. Using the following key, mark the appropriate answer on the answer sheet.

A. Only 1, 2, and 3 are correct
B. Only 1 and 3 are correct
C. Only 2 and 4 are correct
D. Only 4 is correct
E. All are correct

DIRECTIONS SUMMARIZED				
A	B	C	D	E
1,2,3 only	1,3 only	2,4 only	4 only	All are correct

_____ 36. Good practice in coping with clinical problems caused by accidental overdose of methadone is to—

(1) Administer Ipecac if patient is alert and cooperative.
(2) Administer naloxone, but only if the patient becomes hyperactive.
(3) Carry out gastric aspiration and lavage (lavage should be done only by highly experienced ER workers).
(4) Administer naltrexone.

_____ 37. In the emergency diagnosis of a drug overdose, pupillary constriction can be an indication of overdose of—

(1) Ethanol.
(2) Barbiturates.
(3) Phenothiazines.
(4) Narcotics.

_____ 38. Drugs used in treating withdrawal from barbiturates can properly include—

(1) Secobarbital.
(2) Phenobarbital.
(3) Pentobarbital.
(4) Glycopyrrolate.

_____ 39. In cases of tricyclic antidepressant overdose—

   (1) Effects of these drugs are sustained.
   (2) Blood levels of these drugs are easily detectable.
   (3) Experience suggests that physostigmine salicylate can be life-saving.
   (4) Early treatment with stimulant medications is indicated.

_____ 40. With regard to pain management of opiate dependent persons, the following schedule should be applied—

   (1) Methadone maintenance of surgical patients generally takes care of analgesic needs of patients.
   (2) Methadone should be discontinued and meperidine (Demerol) substituted.
   (3) Talwin should be used as an analgesic as it will not interfere with drug maintenance.
   (4) Meperidine (Demerol) should be used in ordinary analgesic doses while the patient is being maintained on methadone.

_____ 41. For the management of methadone maintained patients in the hospital, methadone should be—

   (1) Discontinued and Valium administered 10 mg once a day.
   (2) Administered at usual maintenance levels with once-a-day oral administration.
   (3) Administered orally at doses of 5-10 mg every 8 hours.
   (4) Administered in parenteral doses (where oral administration is not possible) of 5-10 mg every 8 hours.

_____ 42. In the case of the hyperventilating drug abusing patient without other associated medical conditions causing the hyperventilation—

   (1) Oral administration of diazepam (10-20 mg) may prove helpful.
   (2) Larger doses of diazepam may be needed for a patient who is a heavy smoker.

(3) The half-life of the administered diazepam is directly proportionate to the patient's years of age.
(4) Removal of the patient to a quiet, reassuring environment is highly desirable.

_____ 43. Methadone maintenance for pregnant women may be advisable because—

(1) Withdrawal from narcotics may result in fetal death.
(2) Prematurity of the newborn is more common to heroin dependent than methadone maintained mothers.
(3) Patient will otherwise continue to use narcotics, as well as a variety of other drugs.
(4) "Street" heroin use is associated with 80% greater perinatal morbidity and mortality than is methadone maintenance.

_____ 44. Which of the following drugs may be considered to be narcotic antagonists?

(1) Naltrexone.
(2) Cyclazocine.
(3) Naloxone.
(4) Dolophine.

PART V. TRUE-FALSE QUESTIONS

DIRECTIONS: For each statement below, place a check mark next to the "T" if the statement is true, or next to the "F" if it is false.

45. Disulfiram (Antabuse) is always a safe adjunctive therapy for patients who do not continue to drink heavily.

T _____   F _____

46. The most serious problem seen in patients on methadone maintenance is the abuse of barbiturates.

T _____   F _____

47. Clonidine as used in the treatment of opiate withdrawal is usually administered once a day.

T _____   F _____

48. The therapeutic community is the treatment of choice for the less well-motivated drug abuser.

    T _____   F _____

49. Alcoholics Anonymous attempts to provide a crisis response system to provide help to the alcoholic away from home.

    T _____   F _____

50. Physicians are permitted to provide maintenance levels of any opioid drug to opioid dependent patients in a hospital.

    T _____   F _____

TREATMENT POSTTEST ANSWER KEY

Answer	Answer
1. E	26. D
2. E	27. C
3. A	28. B
4. B	29. B
5. E	30. A
6. C	31. B
7. B	32. B
8. C	33. C
9. C	34. B
10. C	35. C
11. A	36. B
12. B	37. D
13. A	38. A
14. B	39. B

TREATMENT POSTTEST ANSWER KEY (continued)

Answer		**Answer**	
15.	C	40.	D
16.	D	41.	C
17.	B	42.	E
18.	A	43.	A
19.	B	44.	A
20.	A	45.	F
21.	A	46.	F
22.	B	47.	F
23.	B	48.	F
24.	C	49.	T
25.	A	50.	F

APPENDIX A
Assessment Interviewing Guide

This appendix is intended to be a guide for the initial interview of the client by the examiner. It suggests certain areas of inquiry and certain kinds of questions that may elicit important information. It can be used as a general guide, but the interview itself should be open-ended so that significant responses can be further used to obtain information of importance that is not asked for directly here. It supplements the routine history and physical examination.

I. READINESS

A. *What brought the client to treatment?*

    1. Family pressure

        a. In what ways has your spouse or family influenced you to seek treatment?

        b. What does your family think about your being here?

    2. Legal pressure

        a. Were you sent here by the courts?

        b. What, if any, legal pressures are bringing you to treatment?

    3. Peer pressure

        a. Have any of your friends been in treatment here?

        b. Have any of your friends been in other treatment programs?

4. Street pressure

    a. Is something happening on the street drug scene that causes you to be here?
    b. Did you come here for reasons of personal safety?

5. Job pressure

    a. Were you sent here by your employer?
    b. If so, what kind of progress do you have to show in treatment in order to keep your job?

6. Medical problems

    a. What medical problems, if any, brought you to treatment now?

7. Internal pressure

    a. Did you decide to come to treatment on your own?
    b. What were the reasons for your decision?

8. Immediacy

    a. What caused you to seek treatment now rather than earlier?
    b. What has changed?

B. *What brought the client to this program?*

1. Preferred modality

    a. What type of treatment do you expect to receive here?

2. Source of information regarding modality

    a. How did you learn about our program?

3. Expectations

    a. What are your expectations regarding the treatment methods used in this program?
    b. Given what you know about the program, what do you anticipate will give you the most difficulty?
    c. How long do you expect that it will take to get straight? (*Or*) How long do you expect to be here?

d. What do you expect it will be like for you next week? Next month? In 6 months?
e. What do you expect you'll be like (regarding behavior) when you are ready to leave treatment?

4. Sources of expectations (personal contact, friends, rumor)

    a. Where do your expectations come from?
    b. What did friends tell you?

5. Attitudes, beliefs, fears

    a. What have you heard about this treatment method?

6. Acceptability

    a. Is this form of treatment acceptable to you?
    b. What other treatment did you consider?

7. Support for client's decision

    a. How do friends (spouse, significant others) feel about your decision?
    b. What things are working against you to prevent treatment?
    c. What things are working for you?

8. Do significant others have an interest in keeping the client dependent?

    a. Who do you think really cares about what happens to you?
    b. How are things and people going to change once you stop using drugs?
    c. What changes do you anticipate in your relationships with your spouse (with others) if you stop using drugs?

C. *Has the client had previous treatment experience?*

1. Previous attempts at treatment

    a. What previous treatment, if any, have you had for drug abuse?

2. Modality

    a. What was the nature of the treatment?

3. Sequence of experiences (if more than one prior experience)

4. Duration

    a. How long did the treatment last?

5. Consequences

    a. What was it like?
    b. What changes did it bring about?

6. Satisfaction

    a. What did you like about the treatment?

7. Dissatisfaction

    a. What did you dislike about the treatment?

8. Reasons for termination

    a. What were the reasons or circumstances for leaving?

9. Who or what was helpful to the client in these programs?

    a. In what way did you find the counselor to be helpful? Not helpful?
    b. What about the experience did you find helpful? Not helpful?
    c. What did you gain from the experience?
    (*If the client gives a negative response, ask*)
    How did you handle it? (*Or*) What did you do with your anger, hostility, disappointment? (*Or whatever client said.*)
    d. What services in the last clinic helped you most? Least?

II. RELATIONSHIPS

A. *Who is (are) the person(s) to whom the client has been closest?*

   1. Quality of the relationship

      a. Tell me about this person.

   2. Feelings about the person and the relationship

      a. How do you feel about this person?
      b. What do you like best about the relationship?
      c. What do you dislike about the relationship, if anything?

   3. Duration of the relationship

      a. How long have you known each other?
      b. How long have you known each other on a close or intimate basis?

   4. Present status

      a. Do you associate with this person now?
      b. Do you keep in touch?
      c. How are you getting along now?

   5. Meaningfulness or depth of relationship

      a. What do you do together?
      b. What do you talk about?
      c. Have you ever told this person things about yourself that no one else knows?
      d. When (or if) you are in trouble, will this person help you out?
      e. How do you handle disagreements?
      f. Are there some secrets that you can trust this person with?
      g. Are there some secrets that you cannot trust this person with?
      h. Are there some things you can depend on this person for? Not depend on him (or her) for?
      i. Can this person trust you?
      j. Can this person depend on you?

B. *What is the quality of the client's relationships with members of the family?*

   1. Specific family members

      (*For all of these, say*) Tell me about your _____.
      a. Mother (natural, foster, step)
      b. Father (natural, foster, step)
      c. Siblings (natural, foster, step)
      d. Other family figures (grandparents, aunts and uncles, godparents, etc.)
      e. Spouse
      f. Children

C. *What was (is) the home like for the client?*

   1. Family

      a. What were some of the positive things you got from your family?
      b. What were some of the negative things you got from your family?
      c. Did your family treat you differently from your brothers or sisters? In what way?
      d. As a child, were there ever times when you wanted to run away from home? Did you? What were the reasons for your leaving?

   2. Adverse family conditions

      a. Drug abuse
      b. Alcoholism
      c. Brutality
      d. Incest or other unusual sexual behaviors (e.g., pedophilia)
      e. Suicide
      f. Mental illness
      g. Compulsive gambling
      h. Compulsive promiscuity
      i. Criminal behviors

3. Unusual family constellations (homosexual or bisexual parents, communal parents, open marriages, etc.)

4. Separation

   a. Have you ever lost someone who meant a lot to you through—
      1. Death
      2. Murder
      3. Suicide
      4. Divorce or separation
      5. Incarceration of brothers, sisters, or parents?
   b. As a child were you ever separated from your family due to—
      1. Illness
      2. Long periods of hospitalization
      3. Other institutionalization (e.g., detention facilities, training schools, etc.)?

D. *Was the client ever separated from his or her family and institutionalized as a child?*

   If the client lived in an institution, inquire about:

   1. Nature of the institution

      a. What kind of an institution or facility was it?

   2. Reasons for placement

      a. Who was responsible for your being in the institution?
      b. Why were you placed there? (*Or*) Why did you choose to go there?
      c. Did you feel your placement there was the right thing for you?
      d. How do you feel about the people responsible for your being there?

   3. Length of confinement

      a. At what age did you enter the facility?
      b. How long did you remain there?

4. The client's attitudes toward the facility and its personnel

   a. What were some of the things that you liked about the facility? Disliked about it?
   b. What were your feelings toward the people who ran the facility?
   c. What people were the most important to you in the institution? In what way did they contribute to your well-being or development?
   d. How would you describe your feelings about institutions in general?

5. Adverse conditions

   a. Drug abuse
   b. Brutality and/or harsh treatment by authorities
   c. Violence on the part of peers
   d. Homosexuality
   e. Physical conditions (poor accommodations, harsh practices, etc.)
   f. Mental illness and/or suicides
   g. Runaway and turnover rates
   h. Relationships with peers (i.e., was client accepted or rejected by peers?)

E. *What is the quality of the client's relationship with members of the same and opposite sex?*

   1. People of the *same* sex

      a. Do you have any male (female) friends?
      b. On the whole, do you like or enjoy being with men (women) more than women (men)?

   2. People of the *opposite* sex

      a. How do you get along with men (women) in general?
      b. Which of the sexes do you get along with better? For what reasons?
      c. With which do you spend the majority of your time?

3. Sexual orientation

   a. What is your major sexual orientation? (Straight, bisexual, gay)
   b. What kind of a person do you prefer as a sexual partner?
   c. How important do you feel sex is in comparison with other aspects of a relationship?

4. Marital status and attitudes

   a. Are you married or living with someone?
      (*If yes*) How do you feel about your marriage (or relationship)?
   b. Have you ever been married (or lived with someone) before? (*If yes*) How many times? What caused the marriage(s) or relationship(s) to end?
   c. What are the things you like about being married (or living with someone)? Dislike?
   d. What do you feel is the most important factor that holds a marriage (or relationship) together? (e.g., love, good sex, getting along well, similarities in taste or temperament, social influences, etc.)

F. *Has the client ever belonged to social or institutional groups?*

1. Membership in special groups
   Have you ever belonged to—

   a. Church groups
   b. Community groups
   c. School groups (extracurricular activities)
   d. Street gangs or social clubs
   e. Political groups
   f. Sports clubs
   g. Military groups
   h. Therapy groups?

   (*If yes for any one or more of the above, inquire about:*)

2. Membership status

   a. How long did you belong to that group?
   b. How often did you attend meetings or get-togethers?

3. Role in group (i.e., leader or follower)

   a. Where did you fit into the group?
   b. What did you do?

4. Extent of group involvement

   a. Did you work cooperatively with others toward a group goal?
   b. Did you pursue your own interests with little interest in activities of other group members?

5. General attitudes toward group affiliations

   a. Do you prefer to spend most of your free time alone, with one other person, or in a group?

III. RATIONALITY

A. *Has the client ever demonstrated extreme mood swings?*

1. Depression

   a. Have you felt really down? What kinds of feelings did you have? (Helpless, hopeless, depressed)
   b. Have you lost your interest or pleasure in things that you usually enjoy?
   c. Have you lost your ability to concentrate?
   d. Have you felt physically down? (Fatigue, headaches, digestive disturbances, etc.)

2. Mania

   a. Have you felt really hyped up—as if your mind or body were speeding?
   b. Has everything seemed really rosy?
   c. Have you gone on binges? (Eating, spending, sex, gambling)

3. Mixed—either depression or mania

   a. Were there changes in your drives or behavior? What kinds of changes?

b. Were there marked changes in your eating habits or in your weight? What kind?

c. Have you had dramatic changes in sleeping patterns? What kinds of changes? (Inability to fall asleep, early morning awakening, no need for sleep)

NOTE: (*If the client answers yes to any of the above, also inquire*) How long did it last? Did it get progressively worse? How were you able to stop it? Is this a problem at this time?

B. *Is the client suicidal?*

1. Suicidal tendencies

   a. Have you ever thought of harming yourself?
   b. Have you ever had thoughts of killing yourself?
   c. Have you feared that you might act on them?
   d. Are you having those fears now or recently?
   e. Is this a problem at this time?

C. *How does the client control strong feeling or impulses?*

1. Impulse control

   a. Can you wait for something, or do you have to have it now?
   b. Do you often act on the spur of the moment without considering the consequences? Give examples.

2. Anger

   a. Do you get angry easily?
   b. What kinds of things make you angry?
   c. How do you handle your anger?
   d. How would I know if you were angry with me?
   e. How do you handle frustration?

3. Driving record

   a. Do you drive?
   b. How often do you drive?
   c. What do you do when other drivers make you angry?
   d. How many times have you been stopped for a moving violation?

4. Food

   a. Have you ever been on a diet?
   b. Were you able to stick to it?

5. Smoking

   a. Do you smoke? (Did you smoke in the past?)
   b. How much do (did) you smoke?
   c. Have you ever tried to quit?
   d. What methods did you use?
   e. What were your reactions?

6. Money

   a. How do you handle money?
   b. Do you budget?
   c. Do you like to gamble?

7. Savings

   a. If you had a 3-day supply of drugs, how long could you make it last?
   b. How do you plan ahead?
   c. When you want something badly, are you able to save up for it?

D. *Does the client have a potential for violence?*

1. Violence potential

   a. Have you ever harmed anyone? (*If yes*) Who was it? What were the circumstances?
   b. Was it when you were drug-free?
   c. Under the influence of drugs?
   d. Would you do it again under similar circumstances? Why or why not?

2. Motivation

   a. Was it survival or self-defense?
   b. Revenge? (NOTE: *Take into consideration data from arrest record, if appropriate.*)

E. *Overall assessment of client's behavior. (See Behavioral Assessment Inventory, page 210.)*

IV. RESOURCES

A. *Is the client employed?*

   1. Nature of the current job (*if employed*)

      a. What kind of work do you do?
      b. How long have you been there?
      c. Do you see yourself staying with this job?
      d. Do you like your co-workers?
      e. Do you see opportunities for advancement?

   2. Previous job history (*if any*)

      a. What kind of work did you do before this?
      b. How long did you work at that job?
      c. Why did you leave?
      d. What did you like about the work there? Dislike?

   3. Nature of work while in jail, military, or similar situations (*if appropriate*). (*Ask questions similar to those in Number 2, above.*)

B. *What kind of job skills does the client have?*

   1. Previous training

      a. What kind of training have you had?
      b. Where was the training received? (Jail, military, vocational program, other)
      c. What did you learn?

   2. Avocational skills and interests

      a. When you were a kid, what kinds of things were you into?
      b. When you were a kid, did you have any hobbies? Do you have any now?

c. What do you like to do?
d. What kinds of things would you like to be able to do?

3. Attitudes toward work

a. If you could write your own ticket, what kind of job would you like to have?
b. What time of day do you work best?
c. Whom do you know who has a good job? Why is it good?

C. *Does the client have job-related competencies?*

1. Hustling behavior

a. Before you came into treatment, how were you raising money for your drugs? (*Straightforward and detailed probing may be required. If the client is evasive, focus on a particular day to serve as an example.*)
b. Where were you involved in the distribution system?
c. What was your source of drugs?

2. Implications of the client's status and income change as a result of entering treatment

a. How will your entering treatment affect your income or the way you earn a living?
b. Will entering treatment affect your status in any other way?

D. *How does the client spend his or her leisure time, relax, have fun?*

1. Current activities

a. Other than drugs, what do you do with your free time?
b. Given that you won't have much money, how would you like to spend your time enjoying yourself?
c. Do you know how you might go about pursuing these interests?
d. Do you know of any places where you might pursue these interests?

2. Relationships with nondrug-abusing individuals

    a. How do you feel about straight people (people who do not abuse drugs)?
    b. Is it difficult for you to talk with these people?
    c. Do you have many straight friends?
    d. Do you know any places where straight people hang out?
    e. Do you ever go there? (*If yes*) How do you feel about going there?

E. *Where does the client live? With whom?*

  1. Duration of current residence

      a. Where do you live?
      b. With whom do you live?
      c. How long have you lived there?

  2. Risks involving current housing

      a. Does your spouse or roommate use drugs?
      b. (*If yes*) How do they feel about your trying to kick?
      c. What things at home make it hard or easy for you to kick?

  3. Satisfaction with or plans to change current housing

      a. What do you like about your present living conditions? Dislike?
      b. Is it dangerous staying where you are presently living? In what way?
      c. What is preventing you from making a change?

  4. Previous residences

      a. Where did you live before this?
      b. How long did you live there?
      c. What has been the longest period of time you lived in any one place?
      d. Do you move often to get away from people or problems?

F. *How far has the client gone in school?*

   1. Degrees and certificates

      a. Do you have any diplomas or certificates from school, or any other training?

   2. Academic performance

      a. What were your grades like?
      b. How did they compare with other students' grades?
      c. How were they with respect to where you wanted to be?
      d. Could you have done better if you wanted to?

   3. Attitudes

      a. What were your feelings about school?
      b. What were some of the things you liked about school? Disliked?

   4. Special interests

      a. Were there any subjects that you really liked?
      b. Were there any subjects in which you got good grades?
      c. Were there any teachers who really turned you on or encouraged you?

   5. Interest in continuing education

      a. Have you ever thought of finishing high school (college) or getting your GED (degree)?
      b. How do you feel about the educational system in general?

   6. Self-education

      a. Do you ever read books or magazines?
      b. (*If yes*) Tell me about something you've read recently or the kinds of things you'd like to read if you had the chance.
      c. Do you take any special interest courses? (e.g., adult education courses, community sports or crafts courses, computer, secretarial, etc.)

G. *Does the client have any medical, dental, hygienic, or nutritional problems that require attention?*

   1. Medical or dental problems

      a. Do you have any medical or dental problems that need immediate attention?

   2. Nutrition

      a. How many meals do you usually eat each day?
      b. Do you eat breakfast? (*If applicable*) Do your children have breakfast before going to school?
      c. What do your children do about lunch at school? (*Buy/take*) Do they have breakfast and lunch every day?
      d. What kinds of foods do you generally eat for your main meals?
      e. Do you feel that you (*and children, if applicable*) are getting enough to eat?
      f. Do you receive any food assistance benefits? (e.g., surplus commodities, food stamps, donated foods, free school lunches)

   3. Children's health (*if applicable*)

      a. Are your children in good health?
      b. Who is responsible for their medical care? (*Specify clinic or private physician*)
      c. What vaccinations have they received? When?
      d. Any serious illnesses or hospitalizations *ever* for any of the children?
      e. Are you concerned about any unusual behavior in your children? (Bedwetting, nightmares, hyperactivity, etc.)
      f. Do you ever give drugs to any of your children for special problems such as sleeplessness, nervousness, or hyperactivity?
      g. Where do you keep your methadone or other drugs in the house? Are they in a child-proof place? (*If applicable*)

Except for Question 4 (which also applies in part to men), the following sections contain questions pertaining to female clients. You are not trying to take a gynecological history here, but simply try-

ing to assess whether or not a medical referral or some basic education is needed.
4. Contraception and gynecological care: knowledge of available techniques—oral contraception, foam, IUD, rhythm method, sterilization of self or spouse

    a. What kind of birth control do you use, if any?
    b. Who takes responsibility for contraception?
    c. When was your last Pap smear? Pelvic examination? What were the results?
    d. Have you ever been treated for pelvic infection? (*If yes*) Which?
    e. Other physical-sexual problems? Specify—venereal diseases, trichomoniasis, fungus infection, urinary problems, painful intercourse, unusual discharge.

5. Pregnancies and abortions

    a. How many pregnancies have you had? Were there any miscarriages or delivery problems? (Caesarean, etc.)
    b. Have you ever had any abortions? What kind? Did you have any medical aftereffects?
    c. What were your feelings about having the abortion? (*If applicable*)
    d. Are you pregnant now? (*If yes*) Are you receiving proper medical care? From whom or where? (*If not under physician's care, make plans for immediate referral.*)

6. Menstrual health

    a. Do you have regular menstrual periods?
    b. Are periods different when you are on or off various drugs?
    c. Do you experience any difficulties (pain, excessive bleeding) with your periods? Is there a difference when you are on or off drugs?

H. *Does the client have a regular source of income?*

1. Source of income (if not covered in employment section)
2. Sufficiency of income
    a. Is your income sufficient to meet your living needs?

3. Money management

    a. Do you have any money in reserve?
    b. Can you hold onto money when you get it or do you spend it right away?
    c. Do you have a bank account?
    d. Where does most of your money go?
    e. Do you like to gamble or play the numbers?
    f. Where do you get your checks cashed?

4. Credit purchases (focus on whether the client loses money because of poor consumer practices)

    a. Do you tend to pay for things right away, or do you make time payments?

5. Debt management (the extent of indebtedness and the client's credit rating)

    a. How do you handle your debts and bills?
    b. What do you think your credit rating is like?

6. Bonding for security jobs

    a. Do you have any interest in security jobs that would require bonding?
    b. Do you think you would have any difficulty getting bonded for security jobs?

BEHAVIORAL ASSESSMENT INVENTORY

To be completed by counselor after the assessment interviews.

Part I: Counselor Observation of the Client's Interview Behavior

1. Behavior:

    Yes   No
    ____ ____   Is he friendly?
    ____ ____   Is he stoned, high, or intoxicated?

___ ___ Is he unusual or different from most clients you have seen?

___ ___ Is he hyper?

___ ___ Is he inactive?

___ ___ Is he alert?

___ ___ Does he initiate conversation?

___ ___ Do you believe him? (Is he credible?)

___ ___ Is he nervous?

___ ___ Does he fidget?

___ ___ Does he sweat?

___ ___ Is he manipulative?

___ ___ Is he seductive?

___ ___ Does he direct the interview?

___ ___ Is he evasive?

___ ___ Is he suspicious?

___ ___ Is he cooperative?

2. Thought Disorder:

   Yes   No

   ___ ___ Does he make sense?

   ___ ___ Is he thinking straight (or rationally)?

   ___ ___ Can you follow him?

   ___ ___ Does his attention wander?

   ___ ___ Does he answer questions appropriately?

   ___ ___ Is the client scared?

3. Sensorium: Does the client know:

Yes   No
___   ___   Time? (Year, month, day of month, day of week)
___   ___   Place? (Geographic location)
___   ___   Person? (His own name)
___   ___   Situation? (The interview or clinic)
___   ___   Is his memory intact? (Recent, remote, recall)

Part II: Counselor's Impression of the Client

Yes   No
___   ___   Do you like the client?
___   ___   Does he scare you?
___   ___   Is he a hustler?
___   ___   Is he a nice person?
___   ___   Does he answer questions superficially, or are his answers substantive?

Prognosis:

_____
_____
_____
_____
_____
_____

General Impressions:

_____

_____

_____

_____

_____

_____

APPENDIX B
Quick Reference Guide to Intoxication, Withdrawal, Overdose, and Emergency Management

This guide is intended as a handy reference to some of the problems found among drug abusing clients. It is not intended to be an exhaustive or detailed examination of problems or of their signs and symptoms.

DRUG AND ALCOHOL OVERDOSE AND THE COMATOSE PATIENT

1. Postpone complete diagnosis until the emergency is less critical.

2. Immediate measures:

    a. If no heartbeat or blood pressure is obtained, external cardiac massage will be required. Ensure an adequate airway, administering oxygen if necessary.
    b. Maintain a rhythmic respiratory rate.
    c. Maintain the cardiovascular system and start intravenous fluids. Vasopressors can be used as needed.
    d. Inject I.V. naloxone (Narcan) 0.4 mg.

3. Once an adequate airway has been established and the cardiovascular system stabilized, attempts should be made to determine what drug(s) the patient has taken.

FEVER OF UNKNOWN ORIGIN IN THE DRUG OR ALCOHOL ABUSER

It is important to determine whether the patient is an intravenous user or exclusively an oral user.

If the patient uses drugs intravenously, consider:

1. Endocarditis—bacterial or fungal
2. "Cotton fever" (the street term for chills and fever following injection of particles or bacteria directly into blood serum)—this is either a bacteremia or foreign-body reaction. The term relates to the cotton sometimes used to filter the injected solution.
3. Drug withdrawal states, especially with depressants
4. Tuberculosis
5. Abscesses anywhere in the body, including organ systems
6. Thrombophlebitis
7. Hepatitis
8. Allergic drug reactions
9. Granulomatous lesions of the lung
10. Pneumonitis

In the nonintravenous user, consider:

1. Alcohol and drug withdrawal states (e.g., delirium tremens)
2. Hepatitis
3. Acute drug reactions
4. Pneumonitis

HELPFUL DIAGNOSTIC AIDS

1. Blood culture
2. Cultures of wounds, drainage, etc.
3. Hepatic enzyme studies
4. Chest X-ray
5. Tubercular skin test
6. Specialized X-ray procedures such as planograms, arteriograms, intravenous pyelograms, or CAT scans.

STIMULANT INTOXICATION AND OVERDOSE

SIGNS	SYMPTOMS	DIAGNOSTIC AIDS
Most common:	*Most common:*	Blood or urine levels of amphetamine or cocaine
Tachycardia	Anorexia	
Hyperpyrexia	Euphoria-Dysphoria	
Diaphoresis	Irritability	
Dilated pupils	Manic affect	
Hypertension	Paresthesia	
Dry mouth	Restlessness	
Tremor	Insomnia	
Hyperactivity	Labile affect	
In higher doses:	*In higher doses or after prolonged use:*	
Delirium	Auditory, visual, and sometimes tactile hallucinations	
Seizures followed by coma		
Hyperactivity	Paranoid ideation or psychosis	
"Overamping"	Stereotyped activity	

STIMULANT WITHDRAWAL

SIGNS	SYMPTOMS	DIAGNOSTIC AIDS
Psychomotor retardation	Aches and pains	Abnormal sleep EEG's
Nasal congestion[1]	General fatigue	Urine screen for cocaine or amphetamines
	Apathy	Depression scales
	Agitation	
	Depression[2]	
	Generalized aches	
	Hyperphagia	
	Hypersomnia	

NOTES: [1] In withdrawal from cocaine when taken by insufflation (snorting).

[2] Because this symptom may be present in other mental disorders, careful clinical evaluation of the psychopathological conditions present before the use of stimulants is important.

HALLUCINOGEN INTOXICATION

SIGNS	SYMPTOMS	DIAGNOSTIC AIDS
Dilated pupils	*Low to moderate doses:*	None are widely available.
Hypertension	Anxiety-elation	Some laboratories can do urine or blood levels. GC with a nitrogen detector or GC-MS instruments are required for those drugs that can produce behavioral changes at blood levels less than 100 ng/ml.
Hyperreflexia	Visual distortions	
Tremor	Hallucinations	
Hyperpyrexia	Changes in body image	
Tachycardia	Labile affect	
Facial flush	Paresthesia	RAI or EMIT for cannabis.
Conjunctival injection (marijuana)	Synesthesias[1]	
	Time-space distortions	
In higher doses:	Rambling speech	
Toxic psychosis	Easy suggestibility	
Seizures (rare)	Anorexia	
Depersonalization	*In higher doses:*	
Paranoid ideation	Acute panic reactions (not necessarily dose related)	

NOTE: [1]The patient may describe "feeling sounds" or "hearing colors."

PHENCYCLIDINE (PCP, ANGEL DUST) INTOXICATION AND OVERDOSE

SIGNS	SYMPTOMS	DIAGNOSTIC AIDS
Low doses: Dysarthria Horizontal and vertical nystagmus Gait ataxia Tachycardia Increased deep tendon reflexes	*Low to moderate doses:* Hyperacusis Floating feeling Aggressiveness Euphoria Analgesia Body distortions Nausea	Blood and urine levels of phencyclidine. Either GC apparatus with a nitrogen detector or GC-MS is required for detection of blood or urine levels in the low nanogram range. Otherwise, false laboratory negatives can confuse the diagnosis. Test may be positive for a week after the last dose.

PHENCYCLIDINE (PCP, ANGEL DUST) INTOXICATION AND OVERDOSE (continued)

SIGNS	SYMPTOMS	DIAGNOSTIC AIDS
Higher doses and overdose:	Amnesia	
Blank stare	*Higher doses:*	
Facial grimaces	Inability to speak	
Hypertension	Labile affect	
Muscle rigidity, spasms	Vomiting	
Seizures	Psychotic reactions, delirium, schizophreniform psychosis	
"Eyes open" coma, levels of consciousness may fluctuate	Paranoid delusions	
Drooling	Hallucinations	

HYPNOSEDATIVE INTOXICATION AND OVERDOSE

SIGNS	SYMPTOMS	DIAGNOSTIC AIDS
Low doses:	*Low doses:*	Blood or urine levels of depressant drugs.
Horizontal and, less frequently, vertical nystagmus	Dizziness	EEG shows a nonspecific slow wave depressant effect.
Dysarthria	Paradoxical excitement or violence	
Ataxia	Confusion	
Depressed respiratory rate	Lethargy, drowsiness	
Hypotension	Clumsiness	
Depressed deep tendon reflexes	*High doses:*	
Stupor	Irritability	
Dysmetria	General sluggishness	
High doses and overdoses:	Inability to concentrate	
Coma		
Shock		
Respiratory arrest		
Pupils may be slightly constricted[1] or unchanged[1]		

NOTE: [1]Except for glutethimide (Doriden), which may be present with dilated pupils or anisocoria.

HYPNOSEDATIVE WITHDRAWAL

SIGNS	SYMPTOMS	DIAGNOSTIC AIDS
Most common: Fever Postural hypotension Diaphoresis Tremors Flushed face Delirium *In severe cases:* Seizures	*Most common:* Anxiety Abdominal cramps Anorexia Irritability Sleeplessness Nightmares *In severe cases:* Gross confusion Hallucinations Shock	EEG showing bursts of spiked, high-amplitude slow waves in non-epileptics[2]

NOTES: [1]Once physical dependence on barbiturates is established, abruptly stopping the drug produces a withdrawal syndrome similar to those for all barbiturates and sedative-hypnotics. The term "depressant withdrawal syndrome" is thus preferred by some authors. The severity of withdrawal depends on the amount and pattern of use and the individual physiological differences of the user. Table 5-1 shows the time-dose required to develop physical dependence to some depressant drugs. Duration of time between cessation of depressant medication and appearance of withdrawal symptoms is related to the half-life of the drug. Alcohol-related withdrawal symptoms usually appear during the first 2 days after withdrawal, while benzodiazepine withdrawal symptoms may not develop until 5 to 7 days after medication is discontinued.

[2]The EEG is of limited diagnostic value within 2 weeks after seizure activity or during drug intoxication.

OPIATE INTOXICATION AND OVERDOSE

SIGNS	SYMPTOMS	DIAGNOSTIC AIDS
Intoxication:	*Low doses:*	Naloxone (Narcan) reverses signs and symptoms of overdose and intoxication
Most common:	Euphoria	Blood or urine levels of opiates
Miosis[1]	Floating feeling	
	Sleepiness	
	Anxiety	
Higher Doses:		
Nodding[2]		
Hypotension		
Hypothermia		
Depressed respirations		
Shock		
Needle marks, tracks		
Cyanosis		
Bradycardia		
Overdoses:		
Pulmonary edema		
Coma		
Apnea		

NOTES: [1] With meperidine (Demerol) the pupils may sometimes be dilated.

[2] The head falls to chest and jerks back several times each minute.

OPIATE WITHDRAWAL

SIGNS	SYMPTOMS[1]	DIAGNOSTIC AIDS
Mild Withdrawal:	Nausea, anorexia	Signs and symptoms are precipitated or intensified by naloxone (Narcan) injection
Yawning	Anxiety	
Dilated pupils	Insomnia	Urine test for opiates or quinine, which may be present 24–48 hours after last dose
In More Severe Cases:	Abdominal cramps	
	Pain in muscles and bones	
Vomiting	Leg spasms "kicking the habit"	
Diarrhea		
Piloerection (gooseflesh)	Irritability	
Rhinorrhea	Restlessness	
Lacrimation	Craving for opiates	
Elevation in pulse rate and blood pressure	Spontaneous ejaculation	

NOTE: [1]"Symptoms usually begin 6 to 12 hours after last use and can last 72 hours or longer depending on the duration of action of the drug used. Methadone withdrawal symptoms develop 12 to 24 hours after last dose and are generally less intense but more prolonged. Withdrawal from Darvon is mild, with onset 6 to 12 hours following last dose. However, withdrawal convulsions have been reported to occur in more severe cases of Darvon withdrawal. Certain minor symptoms can last for several months and are called the "protracted abstinence syndrome."

DRUG SIGNS AND SYMPTOMS

SIGNS & SYMPTOMS	WITHDRAWAL ALCOHOL	WITHDRAWAL STIMULANTS	WITHDRAWAL DEPRESSANTS	WITHDRAWAL OPIATES	INTOXICATION ALCOHOL	INTOXICATION STIMULANTS	INTOXICATION DEPRESSANTS	INTOXICATION OPIATES	INTOXICATION HALLUCINOGENS	INTOXICATION PHENCYCLIDINE	OVERDOSE ALCOHOL	OVERDOSE STIMULANTS	OVERDOSE DEPRESSANTS	OVERDOSE OPIATES	OVERDOSE HALLUCINOGENS	OVERDOSE PHENCYCLIDINE
Abdominal cramps			●	●											●	
Aches, muscle	●	●		●		●										
Affect, labile					●	●			●	●						
Analgesia (pinprick)										●	●	●	●	●		●
Angina												●				
Anorexia	●		●	●	●	●	●	●	●	●		●				●
Anxiety	●	●	●	●	●	●	●	●	●			●			●	●
Arrhythmia						●						●				

	1	2	3	4	5	6	7	8	9	10	11	12	13
Ataxia		●		●		●	●			●	●		●
Body image changes		●				●	●	●		●	●		●
Chest pain							●						
Chills					●							●	
Circulatory collapse		●				●	●						
Coma	●	●			●	●	●						
Comprehension, slow	●	●				●	●						
Convulsions	●	●					●						
Coryza					●								
Delirium	●				●	●	●	●	●	●	●	●	●
Depressed mood						●	●				●		
Diarrhea							●	●		●		●	●
Diplopia					●		●	●		●			
Dizziness		●			●	●		●		●			
Dysmetria	●					●		●					

DRUG SIGNS AND SYMPTOMS (continued)

SIGNS & SYMPTOMS	WITHDRAWAL ALCOHOL	WITHDRAWAL STIMULANTS	WITHDRAWAL DEPRESSANTS	WITHDRAWAL OPIATES	INTOXICATION ALCOHOL	INTOXICATION STIMULANTS	INTOXICATION DEPRESSANTS	INTOXICATION OPIATES	INTOXICATION HALLUCINOGENS	INTOXICATION PHENCYCLIDINE	OVERDOSE ALCOHOL	OVERDOSE STIMULANTS	OVERDOSE DEPRESSANTS	OVERDOSE OPIATES	OVERDOSE HALLUCINOGENS	OVERDOSE PHENCYCLIDINE
Euphoria					●	●	●	●	●	●						
Facial grimacing										●		●				
Fatigue	●	●	●	●												
Floating feeling					●		●	●	●	●						
Flushing	●		●		●		●	●	●		●	●			●	
Hallucinations			●			●			●	●	●	●	●		●	●
Headaches			●									●				
Hyperphagia		●							●							

226

Symptom	1	2	3	4	5	6	7	8	9	10	11	12	13	14	15	16
Hypertension	•	•					•			•	•	•				•
Hyperthermia	•	•		•			•	•		•						•
Hypotonia			•	•								•				
Irritability			•	•						•	•					
Lacrimation	•	•		•			•	•		•			•			•
Memory, poor											•					•
Motor seizures (grand mal)	•			•		•	•		•	•	•					•
Mouth dry	•	•								•			•			
Muscle spasms (rigidity)			•													
Nausea				•	•		•				•	•				•
Nystagmus	•	•		•		•	•			•			•			
Orthostatic hypotension	•	•		•		•	•			•	•					•
Paresthesia					•		•									
Piloerection (gooseflesh)																
Psychosis (toxic)	•	•		•			•			•						•

DRUG SIGNS AND SYMPTOMS (continued)

SIGNS & SYMPTOMS	WITHDRAWAL				INTOXICATION						OVERDOSE					
	ALCOHOL	STIMULANTS	DEPRESSANTS	OPIATES	ALCOHOL	STIMULANTS	DEPRESSANTS	OPIATES	HALLUCINOGENS	PHENCYCLIDINE	ALCOHOL	STIMULANTS	DEPRESSANTS	OPIATES	HALLUCINOGENS	PHENCYCLIDINE
Pupils–dilated				●		●			●			●			●	
Pupils–pinpoint								●						●		
Reflexes, hyperactive	●	●	●			●			●	●		●			●	●
Respiration, slow and shallow											●		●	●		
Restlessness	●	●	●	●		●				●						
Rhinorrhea		●		●												
Skin picking						●		●				●				
Sleep disturbance	●	●	●	●	●	●			●			●				

	Sleepiness	Speech, slurred	Stare, blank	Suspiciousness	Sweating	Tachycardia	Talkativeness	Tremor	Violence	Vomiting	Yawning
			●	●		●			●		
				●		●		●		●	
									●	●	
				●	●	●	●	●		●	
						●			●	●	●
			●	●	●		●			●	●
				●		●		●			
	●										
	●	●		●					●		●
				●		●	●	●	●		
	●	●		●			●		●	●	●
					●	●				●	●
						●		●	●		
					●	●		●	●	●	

APPENDIX C
Resources for Training the Physician and Health Professional in Drugs, Alcohol, and Prescribing: An Annotated Compendium

INTRODUCTION

The *Compendium* is a concise description of education resources on drugs, alcohol, and the problem of prescribing for the medical and health professions educator. Part 1 is a synopsis of drug and alcohol education resources. The first four sections describe materials immediately useful for teaching: curricula and general reviews of education resources (1–17), clinical manuals (18–26), films and videocassettes (27–35), and examinations and certification procedures (36–38). The fifth section has information on organizations that are sources of research or clinical data or from which new education resources may be obtained (39–45).

Part 2 presents information on the problem of prescribing, dispensing, and administering controlled substances. Section one is a description of texts and organizational resources from which information may be obtained on the problem of proper prescribing in general (46–52); prescribing for specific indications such as sleep disturbance (53–56), pain (57), and the elderly (58); or on issues to be considered in alcohol and prescribing (22 and 26). Section two presents resources on the problem of diversion of drugs for purposes of abuse (59–68). Resources for information on the general problem of diversion and measures to address the problem (59–61) and resources for physicians (62–64), pharmacists (65–67), and hospital personnel (68) are described. Section three presents materials and programs to address the

231

problem of the impaired physician (69–72, 78), pharmacist (73–74), nurse (75–76), and dentist (77). Section four describes state-wide education or enforcement programs (79–90) and gives information on an American Medical Association manual, which outlines procedures for establishing state-wide education programs on prescribing and diversion (91).

Each entry of the *Compendium* identifies the audience(s) for which the resource was primarily developed, gives information on where the resource may be obtained, specifies the nature of the resource, and provides a synopsis of its content.

MEDICAL AND HEALTH PROFESSIONS EDUCATION IN DRUGS AND ALCOHOL

Specializing in teaching drugs and alcohol is a recent phenomenon in the history of medical and health professions education. Yet just as it would be unthinkable to remove oncology or cardiology from today's medical school curricula, so in the next generation it may be equally untenable to consider not teaching drugs and alcohol. The same may be true in the teaching of the other health professions as well. To provide a context in which to understand how several of the curriculum resources were developed, we will sketch the history of the development of the field of drug and alcohol education.

Within the present century there has been a growing interest in the treatment of drug and alcohol abuse and dependence. Moral condemnation and punitive approaches often predominated in earlier years. But within the past 25 years a growing understanding of the nature of dependence, the emergence of the disease model concept of dependence, and the development of pharmacologic and social treatment resources have led to a more enlightened approach to treatment (Austin, 1978; DuPont, Goldstein, and O'Donnell, 1979; Kissin and Begleiter, 1971–1983).

Teaching of drugs and alcohol, however, was not conducted in a systematic widespread manner until the early 1970's. In 1970, the National Council on Alcoholism conducted a conference to review the status of training in alcoholism. The conference report highlighted the fact that although alcoholism is a major source of medical pathology and a leading public health problem, teaching in alcoholism was neglected in medical schools (Seixas and Sutton, 1971). In 1972, the Josiah Macy Jr. Foundation (1973) conducted a conference on the problem of substance abuse teaching. Experts were invited to represent the basic sciences and clinical departments of medical schools, federal and state government agencies, professional associations, and pharmaceutical companies. The conferees stressed the need to educate physicians and develop leaders in the drug and alcohol education field. A model curriculum was recommended. The American Medical Association (AMA) Council on Mental Health (1972) expressed its concern about the problem and issued a position paper stressing the need for education and outlining the areas that a curriculum should address.

In 1971, the National Institute on Drug Abuse (NIDA) and the National Institute on Alcohol Abuse and Alcoholism (NIAAA) initiated a program to establish a curriculum in drug abuse and alcoholism in each U.S. medical school, develop the institutional capacity in schools to teach medical students to diagnose and treat persons suffering from substance abuse, and provide medical students and doctors with an understanding of and an ability to properly prescribe licitly manufactured drugs.

NIDA and NIAAA invited each school of medicine, osteopathy, and public health to apply for a grant to train a senior member of the faculty for a career in teaching drugs and alcohol. The "Career Teacher" proposed a plan for his or her training in the addictions and for educating medical students in drugs and alcohol. A total of 60 Career Teacher Grants were awarded. In addition, two Career Teacher Training Centers were established to provide training to Career Teachers and other medical school faculty in educational methodologies and the diagnosis and treatment of addictive disorders. The Career Teacher Training Centers also hosted quarterly meetings of the Career Teachers and served as a locus for knowledge development in medical education.

From the inception of the program, there was a concerted effort to create a collegial atmosphere among all those involved. The Career Teachers, representatives of NIDA and NIAAA, and Training Center Faculty met three times a year to receive training from persons knowledgeable in the field; collaborate in the development of curricula and educational products; and develop programs to inform students, faculty, and practitioners about recent developments in the field of drugs and alcohol. Several substantive undertakings resulted from this activity.

Clinical monographs, *The Medical Monograph Series*, were published on the diagnosis and treatment of drugs and alcohol, on the pharmacology and toxicology of abused drugs, and on prescribing. Drug and alcohol examinations were developed by a task force appointed by the National Board of Medical Examiners and are available for administration by faculty in all U.S. medical schools. Third, the Association of Medical Education and Research in Substance Abuse (AMERSA) was formed. Membership is open to all medical educators and researchers in substance abuse. AMERSA's objectives are to foster the exchange of ideas and develop teaching programs for translating research findings into drug and alcohol curricula. AMERSA members represent approximately 75 medical schools.

Fourth, a Health Professions Education Task Force was formed in 1974 and again in 1978. The Task Force was established because of a realization that osteopaths, nurses, psychologists, pharmacists, physicians' assistants, and social workers had not received adequate education and training in substance abuse. Each of these professions were represented on the Task Force. The Task Force's Committee on Licensure and Certification collaborated with representatives of six medical specialty licensing boards and with the Nursing, Osteopath, Psychology, Social Work, Physician Assistant, and Pharmacy Boards to develop drug and alcohol questions for certifying and licensing examinations. The Committee on Professional Education conducted and published surveys on drug and alcohol education in the professional schools and worked with representatives of each of the national professional associations to develop education materials and programs for the professions.

Next, the Health Professions Education (HPE) program was established at the NIAAA National Clearinghouse for Alcohol Information. The objective of the program is to encourage health professions educators to incorporate comprehensive instruction on alcohol and drug abuse into the preclinical and clinical curricula of physicians, nurses, nurse practitioners, psychologists, and social workers. The HPE project has three major activities: the expansion of a data base of accessible information for course preparation; the development and dissemination of current information, curriculum guides, and other teaching resources; and the fostering of the use of the guides through collaboration with the professional associations and other intermediary organizations.

Next, as an aid to faculty developing drug and alcohol curricula, the Substance Abuse Librarians Information Service (SALIS) was developed. SALIS is an international organization of directors of libraries and resource centers that have large collections of alcohol and drug materials. SALIS' goal is to systematize referencing and loaning procedures and thereby provide better service to persons seeking substance abuse information.

In November 1982, the first international conference on medical education in alcohol and drug abuse was held in Oakland, California. The conference was sponsored by AMERSA and the World Health Organization (WHO). Cosponsors were NIDA, NIAAA, and the Addiction Research Foundation of Toronto, Canada.

Most recently, the State of California has begun to certify physicians to practice in drugs and alcohol. Also, several professional organizations, including the American Academy of Addictionology, the American Medical Association, the California Society for the Treatment of Alcoholism and Other Drug Dependencies, the American Medical Society on Alcoholism, the National Institute on Drug Abuse, and the National Institute on Alcohol Abuse and Alcoholism, and others convened meetings to discuss procedures for national certification and the development of a subspecialty in substance abuse. Currently, the American Medical Society on Alcoholism and Other Drug Dependencies has accepted responsibility for pursuing this.

In summarizing the findings of his 1981 survey on drug abuse and alcoholism teaching in medical schools, Pokorny (1983) concludes that while "during the five year period of 1976–1981, there was a notable improvement in several areas related to alcohol and drug abuse teaching in medical schools," when compared with the results of his 1976 survey (Pokorny, 1978), the percentage of required hours still remains below 1%. He attributes much of the increase in teaching to the presence of Career Teachers in medical schools and to the effect of the Career Teacher Training Program activities in medical education in general. He notes, however, that the amount of time given to teaching drugs and alcohol is still "far out of proportion to the prevalence and importance of alcoholism and drug abuse in public health and in hospital and office practice" (320–321).

PRESCRIBING

Early in the 1970's, the Drug Enforcement Administration (DEA) became concerned about the problem of the diversion of licitly prescribed drugs for the purposes of misuse. In keeping with its responsibilities for administering the Controlled Substances Act, the DEA initiated a major campaign to educate members of the health professions through its Voluntary Compliance Program. Through regional conferences, the publication of guidelines, and the development of programs with professional schools and associations, the DEA educated members about proper prescribing practices and the safeguards required to reduce the problem of diversion.

In 1980, the White House Conference on Prescribing brought together representatives of the medical and other health professions, the regulatory and enforcement community, the pharmaceutical industry, and federal and state health agencies. It focused attention on the need for a coordinated approach to the problem and set in motion, through the AMA, an effective process for doing this.

In 1981 the AMA established the Informal Steering Committee on Prescription Drug Abuse with over 20 organizations representing prescribers, dispensers, manufacturers, regulators, and enforcement agencies. Through its subcommittees, the Steering Committee has developed educational materials for members of the professions and for the consumer. It has also cosponsored state and regional meetings with state medical and other health professional societies, regulatory and health agencies, DEA, and NIDA. The Steering Committee and those who collaborate with its leaders and members comprise the single most knowledgeable and active group in the field of prescribing.

CONCLUSION

Many of the resources in the *Compendium* are the results of the efforts described above. Of course, several products come from other sources. While there are other streams of activity that contribute to the development of the field, it is beyond the scope of this paper to describe these in detail. We have described the development of a new field in which we worked extensively with our federal coworkers and members of the medical and health professions communities for the past 10 years.

The *Compendium* is intended as a resource to the medical and health professions educators. Our hope is that persons and their families who are struggling with the problem of drugs and alcohol and the members of the professions assisting them may find the help and information that they need.

REFERENCES

American Medical Association Council on Mental Health. Medical education on abuse of alcohol and other psychoactive drugs. *Journal of the American Medical Association*, 1972, *219*, 1746-59.

Austin, G.A. *Perspectives on the history of psychoactive substance use.* NIDA Research Issues No. 24, ADAMHA Publication No. 179-810. Washington, D.C.: U.S. Government Printing Office, 1978.

DuPont, R.L., Goldstein, A., and O'Donnell (Eds.). *Handbook on drug abuse.* Washington, D.C.: U.S. Government Printing Office, 1979.

Josiah Macy, Jr., Foundation. *Medical education in drug abuse: Report of a Macy conference.* Philadelphia: William F. Fell, 1973.

Kissin, B., and Begleiter, H. (Eds.). *The biology of alcoholism* (7 vols.). New York: Plenum Press, 1971-1983.

Pokorny, A., Putnam, P., and Fryer, J. Drug abuse and alcoholism teaching in medical and osteopathic schools. *Journal of Medical Education*, 1978, *52*, 816-824.

Pokorny, A., and Solomon, J. A follow-up survey on drug abuse and alcoholism teaching in medical schools. *Journal of Medical Education*, 1983, *58*, 316-321.

Seixas, F.A., and Sutton, J.Y. (Eds.). Professional training on alcoholism. *Annals of the New York Academy of Sciences*, 1971, *178*, 1-139.

PART I:

DRUG AND ALCOHOL EDUCATION RESOURCES

Section One: Curricula and General Reviews of Education Resources (1–17)

(1)

Audience Medical educators
Health professions educators

Further Information National Clearinghouse for Alcohol Information
P.O. Box 2345
Rockville, Maryland 20852
(301) 468-2600

Resource: Curriculum objectives

Physician education in substance abuse: Curriculum objectives. Rockville, Maryland: National Institute on Alcohol Abuse and Alcoholism, and National Institute on Drug Abuse, 1979.

The objectives were prepared in 1979 by a Career Teacher committee of medical school faculty in drugs and alcohol. The objectives are principal areas that should be taught on substance abuse.

(2)

Audience Family physicians

Further Information Society of Teachers of Family Medicine
1740 West 92nd Street
Kansas City, Missouri 64114
(800) 821-2512

Resource: Curriculum

Liepman, M. R., Anderson, R. C., and Fisher, J. V. (Eds.). *Family medicine curriculum guide to substance abuse.* Kansas City, Missouri: Society for Teachers of Family Medicine, 1984.

This curriculum is for teachers of family medicine residents. It contains an extensive annotated list of books, films, and other education resources.

(3)

Audience   Psychiatry faculty

Further Information   National Clearinghouse for Alcohol Information
                         P.O. Box 2345
                         Rockville, Maryland 20852
                         (301) 468-2600

Resource: Curriculum guide

Gallant, D. S. *Alcohol and drug abuse curriculum guide for psychiatry faculty.* Rockville, Maryland: National Clearinghouse for Alcohol Information, 1982.

The monograph is a guide for psychiatric and other medical faculty in teaching alcohol and drug dependence to medical students. The guide explains and summarizes the core material most important for the student to learn, and contains a list of curriculum materials and a selected bibliography.

(4)

Audience   Nurse practitioner faculty

Further Information   National Clearinghouse for Alcohol Information
                         P.O. Box 2345
                         Rockville, Maryland 20852
                         (301) 468-2600

Resource: Curriculum guide

Hasselblad J. *Alcohol abuse curriculum guide for nurse practitioner faculty.* Rockville, Maryland: National Clearinghouse for Alcohol Information, 1984.

This guide covers three areas of instruction: recognition, diagnosis, and management. It is for nurse practitioner faculty who do not have expertise in alcohol education, but who desire to introduce alcohol instruction into their curricula. The core content is presented in outline form and is supported by recommended texts, background readings, and teaching methodologies. It is presumed that students will already have completed a generic nursing program and possess history-taking, physical assessment, and clinical decision-making skills. In Part Three, strategies for mobilization and intervention, available treatment methods, problems encountered in recovery, and family needs are presented.

(5)

Audience   Medical and osteopathic school faculty

Further Information   National Clearinghouse for Alcohol Information
P.O. Box 2345
Rockville, Maryland 20852
(301) 468-2600

Resource: Curriculum guide

Hostetler J. R. *Alcohol and drug abuse teaching methodology guide for medical faculty.* Rockville, Maryland: National Clearinghouse for Alcohol Information, 1982.

The guide is for instructors in medical and osteopathic schools. It presents a variety of new approaches for teaching substance abuse disorders, reviews effective instructional methodologies, and recommends resources useful for developing alcohol and drug curricula.

(6)

Audience   Behavioral science faculty
Health professions educators

Further Information   National Clearinghouse for Alcohol Information
P.O. Box 2345
Rockville, Maryland 20852
(301) 468-2600

Resource: Literature review

Krug, R. S. *Research review of alcohol and drug abuse for behavioral sciences faculty* (RPO-370). Rockville, Maryland: National Clearinghouse for Alcohol Information, 1981.

Based on a survey of literature published between 1976 and 1980, this paper delineates and discusses some major issues in drug and alcohol dependence dealt with in the behavioral sciences.

(7)

Audience	Medical students
	Osteopathic medicine students
	Health professions educators
Further Information	National Clearinghouse for Alcohol Information
	P.O. Box 2345
	Rockville, Maryland 20852
	(301) 468-2600

Resource: Curriculum guide

Gastfriend, D. R. *Obtaining a medical education in alcohol and drug dependence: A student's guide* (RPO-371). Rockville, Maryland: National Clearinghouse for Alcohol Information, 1981.

This paper discusses the need to educate medical students about drugs and alcohol, outlines a curriculum to meet that need, and suggests ways for medical students to obtain training in this field.

(8)

Audience	Medical educators
Further Information	Office of Academic Affairs
	Veterans Administration Central Office
	141-B
	Washington, D.C. 20420
	(202) 389-5171

Resource: Compendium of education resources

A guide for physician training in substance abuse. Washington, D.C.: Veterans Administration, 1983.

The guide reviews drug and alcohol education resources (texts, articles, audiovisuals, and organizations) that may be used to educate physicians in ten skill areas (history taking, physical examination, diagnosis, treatment, prevention, teaching, clinical management, leadership, research, and laboratory testing).

(9)

Audience	Medical educators
	Health professional educators

Further Information   National Clearinghouse for Alcohol Information
P.O. Box 2345
Rockville, Maryland 20852
(301) 468-2600

Resource: Annotated references

Annotated reference list on alcohol and substance abuse for medical educators (RPO-306). Dartmouth University: Project Cork, 1980.

An extensive list of general texts, handbooks, journals, and newsletters on drug and alcohol dependence. Topics covered include education, basic sciences, economics, sociology, etiology, medical consequences, and treatment of alcoholism and substance abuse.

(10)

Audience   Health professions educators

Further Information   National Clearinghouse for Alcohol Information
P.O. Box 2345
Rockville, Maryland 20852
(301) 468-2600

Resource: Journal abstracts

Lyons-Callahan, C.M. *Medical abstracts for educators in alcohol and drug abuse* (RPO-308). Rockville, Maryland: National Clearinghouse for Alcohol Information, 1982.

An annotated bibliography of approximately 100 recent (1975–1982) articles and conference papers on treatment, curricula, and attitudes. Author(s), title, journal, pages, and year are cited.

(11)

Audience   Health professionals

Further Information   (See below.)

Resource: Journal review

Andrews, T., and Cohen, S. Subject journal review: Drug and alcohol abuse periodicals. *Behavioral and Social Sciences Librarian*, 1979, 1, 59–77.

A review of substance abuse periodicals.

(12)
Audience	Librarians
	Health professions educators
Further Information	Addiction Research Foundation
	Marketing Division
	33 Russell Street
	Toronto, Ontario
	M5S 2S1 CANADA
	(807) 595-6000

Resource: Book review index

Bemko, J. *Substance abuse book review index.* Toronto: Addiction Research Foundation, 1984.

The index has appeared annually since 1979, covering materials published since 1978 in 250 journals. It indexes reviews by author, editor, title, and subject, and cites the journal volume, issue, pages, and date. The names of reviewers are included.

(13)
Audience	Health professionals
	Lay public
Further Information	National Clearinghouse for Alcohol Information
	P.O. Box 2345
	Rockville, Maryland 20852
	(301) 468-2600

Resource: Report to Congress

Alcohol and health: Fifth special report to the U.S. Congress from the Secretary of Health and Human Services. Rockville, Maryland: National Institute on Alcohol Abuse and Alcoholism, 1983.

Alcohol and health is a comprehensive review of research and social indicators in the alcohol field. The report reviews the epidemiologic data, genetics, psychobiology, medical consequences, effects on pregnancy, adverse social consequences, treatment, and prevention of alcohol abuse and alcoholism.

(14)
Audience	Librarians
	Health professions educators

Further Information   Ms. Andrea Mitchell
                             Alcohol Research Group
                             1816 Scenic Avenue
                             Berkeley, California 94709
                             (415) 642-5208

Resource: Librarian organization/directory

SALIS, Substance Abuse Librarians and Information Specialists, is an association of persons working in library and information services dealing with alcohol, tobacco, and other psychoactive drugs. SALIS publishes an annual *Directory* on substance abuse information and services available from approximately 100 libraries and information centers in Australia, Canada, England, Finland, Mexico, the Netherlands, New Zealand, Sweden, Switzerland, the United States, and Yugoslavia.

(15)
Audience   Librarians
                             Health professions educators

Further Information   Ms. Theodora Andrews
                             Librarian
                             Purdue University Pharmacy,
                                Nursing and Health Sciences Library
                             Pharmacy Building
                             Purdue University
                             West Lafayette, Indiana 47907
                             (313) 494-1417

Resource: Bibliographies/resources

Ms. Andrews compiles and publishes bibliographies and annotated lists of resources for substance abuse educators and librarians.

(16)
Audience   Health professions educators

Further Information   National Clearinghouse for Alcohol Information
                             P.O. Box 2345
                             Rockville, Maryland 20852
                             (301) 468-2600

Resource: Journal

Health professions education. *Alcohol Health and Research World*, 1983 8(2), 2–36.

This special issue on health professions education describes education programs for physicians, physicians' assistants, pharmacists, nurses, dentists, and social workers. The journal is produced quarterly by the National Institute on Alcohol Abuse and Alcoholism through the Clearinghouse.

(17)
Audience	Health professionals
	Lay public
Further Information	Health and Human Behavior Program
	American Medical Association
	535 North Dearborn Street
	Chicago, Illinois 60610
	(312) 645-5067

Resource: Annotated bibliography

Bibliography of patient and public educational resources on prescription drug abuse. Chicago, Illinois: American Medical Association, 1985.

The bibliography describes education materials available to health professionals and the public on prescription drug abuse. It also contains an extensive index referencing materials by audience, format, and language.

Section Two: Clinical Manuals (18–26)

(18)
Audience	Physicians
Further Information	(Publisher)

Resource: Chapter

Jaffe, J. H. Drug addiction and drug abuse. In A. G. Gilman, L. S. Goodman, and A. Gilman (Eds.). *The pharmacological basis of therapeutics* (6th Ed.). New York: Macmillan, 1980.

This chapter discusses definitions and terminology, genesis of drug use and dependence, clinical characteristics of drugs used for subjective purposes, treatment, the role of the medical profession in prevention of dependence, and the impact of legislation and societal attitudes on patterns and treatment of drug abuse.

(19)
Audience   Physicians
                        Nurses
                        Psychologists

Further Information   (Publisher)

Resource: Book

Kissin, B., and Begleiter, H. (Eds.). *The biology of alcoholism* (7 vols.). New York: Plenum Press, 1971–1983. Vol. 1. Biochemistry (1971). Vol. 2. Physiology and Behavior (1972). Vol. 3. Clinical Pathology (1974). Vol. 4. Social Agents of Alcoholism (1976). Vol. 5. Treatment and Rehabilitation of the Chronic Alcoholic (1977). Vol. 6. The Pathogenesis of Alcoholism: Psychosocial Factors (1983). Vol. 7. The Pathogenesis of Alcoholism: Biological Factors (1983).

This work presents a "comprehensive description of the complex interaction of the chemical substance alcohol with man and with human society" (vol. 2, p. viii).

(20)
Audience   Physicians

Further Information   National Clearinghouse for Drug Abuse Information
                        P.O. Box 416
                        Kensington, Maryland 20895
                        (301) 443-6500

Resource: Monographs

Clinical monographs in the *Medical monograph series* have been published on the diagnosis and treatment of drugs and alcohol, the pharmacology and toxicology of abused drugs, and prescribing. Single copies are available. Titles of the series are:

Senay, E. C., Becker, C. E., and Schnoll, S. H. *Emergency treatment of the drug abusing patient for treatment staff physicians*. Rosslyn, Virginia: National Drug Abuse Center, 1977.

Inaba, D., Way, E. L., Blum, K., and Schnoll, S. H. *Pharmaco-*

logical and toxicological perspectives of commonly abused drugs. Rosslyn, Virginia: National Drug Abuse Center, 1978.

Cohen, S., and Gallant, D. M. *Diagnosis of drug and alcohol abuse.* Brooklyn, New York: Career Teacher Center, SUNY Downstate, 1981.

Senay, E. C., Raynes, A. E., Becker, C. E., and Schnoll, S. H. *The primary physician's guide to drug abuse treatment.* Brooklyn, New York: Career Teacher Center, SUNY Downstate, 1979.

Cohen, S., Buchwald, C., Solomon, J., Callahan, J., and Katz, D. (Eds.). *Frequently prescribed and abused drugs.* Brooklyn, New York: Career Teacher Center, SUNY Downstate, 1980. (This volume is also available for purchase from The Haworth Press, New York.)

Lewis, D. C., and Senay, E. C. *Treatment of drug and alcohol abuse.* Brooklyn, New York: Career Teacher Center, SUNY Downstate, 1981.

(21)
Audience   Physicians
                     Health professionals

Further Information   Vista Hill Foundation
                        3420 Camino del Rio North, Suite 100
                        San Diego, California 90108
                        (619) 563-1770

Resource: Newsletter

Cohen, S. (Ed.). *Drug abuse and alcoholism newsletter.* San Diego, California: Vista Hill Foundation.

The newsletter is published ten times a year and is distributed on a complimentary basis as part of the Foundation's continuing education program. The newsletter presents clear and concise discussions of pharmacologic, clinical, social, legal, and ethical issues on legal and illegal dependence-producing drugs.

(22)
Audience   Physicians
                     Health professionals

Further Information   (Publisher)

Resource: Book

Cohen, S. *The substance abuse problem.* New York: The Haworth Press, 1981.

The book is in five chapters. The first chapter describes the abuse of many legal and illegal drugs and details the effects of that abuse. The second chapter analyzes the trends in drug abuse and relates the global nature of the problem. The third and fourth chapters describe the diagnosis and treatment of certain abuse problems. Chapter five is a discussion of special situations and groups in the abuse of drugs.

(23)
Audience   Physicians

Further Information   American Medical Association
                            Order Department
                            P.O. Box 10946
                            Chicago, Illinois 60610

Resource: Book

Wilford, B. B. *Drug abuse: A guide for the primary care physician.* Chicago, Illinois: American Medical Association, 1981.

The book presents a comprehensive view of drug abuse for the primary care physician. The first section discusses definitions and the etiology of drug abuse, major drugs of abuse, trends in drug abuse, and physician attitudes. Section two contains chapters on screening for drug abuse in a general patient population, care of acute drug reactions, chemical complications, and rehabilitation. The final section discusses legal considerations, prescribing, the drug abusing physician, and prevention and early intervention.

(24)
Audience   Physicians
                            Osteopaths
                            Nurses
                            Physician assistants

Further Information   Addiction Research Foundation
                            Marketing Services
                            33 Russell Street
                            Toronto, Canada M5S 15
                            (807) 595-6000

Resource: Treatment manual

Diagnosis and treatment of alcoholism for primary care physicians. Toronto: Alcoholism and Drug Addiction Research Foundation, 1978.

(25)
Audience   Physicians
                      Osteopaths
                      Nurses
                      Physician assistants

Further Information American Medical Association
                      Order Department
                      P.O. Box 10946
                      Chicago, Illinois 60610

Resource: Treatment manual

Manual on alcoholism (3rd ed.). Chicago, Illinois: American Medical Association, 1977.

(26)
Audience   Physicians
                      Health professionals

Further Information (Publisher)

Resource: Book

Cohen, S. *The alcoholism problem.* New York: The Haworth Press, 1983.

"The current issues and controversies about beverage alcohol and its potential disorders have been selected for consideration in this volume. Not all of the short essays are problem oriented. Some were written because new and pertinent knowledge has recently come forth" (Preface). The book is in three parts: The Nature of Alcohol, The Nature of Alcoholism, and Alcohol/Drug Relationships.

Section Three: Films and Videocassettes (27–35)

(27)
Audience   Health professionals

Further Information Addiction Research Foundation
                      33 Russell Street
                      Toronto, Ontario M5S 2S1
                      (807) 595-6000

Resources: Monographs, films

The Addiction Research Foundation sells educational materials, including pamphlets, fact sheets, books, and audiovisuals. The Foundation publishes two periodicals: *The Journal* and *Projection* (film and video review service). An *Educational Materials Catalogue* is also available.

(28)
Audience	Physicians
Further Information	*Sale*: Operation Cork
	8939 Villa La Jolla Drive
	San Diego, California 92037
	(714) 452-5716
	Rent: Modern Talking Picture Service
	5000 Park Street North
	St. Petersburg, Florida 33709
	(813) 541-7571

Resource: Films/study guides

Four clinical teaching films demonstrate techniques in diagnosis and referral:

Attitudes. 22 min.; 16 mm; color.
Early diagnosis. 20 min.; 16 mm; color.
Confirming the diagnosis/initiating treatment. 13 min.; 16 mm; color.
The physician's role in rehabilitation. 20 min.; 16 mm; color.
CME Category I is available; study guide is necessary.

(29)
Audience	Health professionals
Further Information	Director
	Documentaries for Learning
	Harvard Medical School
	58 Fenwood Road
	Boston, Massachusetts 02115

Resource: Film

Born with a habit. 1971; 30 min.; 16 mm; color.

A number of physiological, psychological, and social problems are associated with the birth of children to narcotic-addicted mothers. This film is recommended to help medical students understand the attitudes of women with addicted babies, as well as the attitudes of health care professionals.

(30)
Audience   Physicians
                        Nurses

Further Information   Eli Lilly and Company
                        Indianapolis, Indiana 46206

Resource: Film

Treatment of acute drug overdose. 1972; 32 min.; 16 mm; color.
   The film describes in detail techniques for emergency treatment of drug overdose victims.

(31)
Audience   Health professionals

Further Information   Operation Cork
                        P.O. Box 9550
                        San Diego, California

Resource: Film

Soft is the heart of a child. 1978; 20 min.; 16 mm; color.
   Demonstrates the effects of alcoholism on the family. Family violence and child abuse and neglect are depicted. An alcoholic father convinces his wife to join him in drinking. The film illustrates such themes as the family consequences of drinking, community paralysis, women as battered spouses and drinkers, children as victims and emissaries to the community, the role of the school, and enabling.

(32)
Audience   Health professionals

Further Information   The Johnson Institute
                        10700 Olson Memorial Highway
                        Minneapolis, Minnesota 55441

Resource: Film

The enablers. 1978; 23 min.; 16 mm; color.
The intervention. 1978; 28 min.; 16 mm; color.

A two-part series. *The enablers* depicts the well-intentioned behavior of family, friends, and a supervisor that helps an alcoholic mother-wife-employee-neighbor to continue her drinking. Each person close to the woman suffers yet seems unable to break out of a self-defeating pattern of interaction; each person is shown undermining the efforts of the other to gain control over the woman's problem. The film demonstrates the dynamics of the chemically dependent family.

In *The intervention*, the husband joins forces with the supervisor to gather together family and friends for coercive, constructive confrontation of an alcoholic wife-mother-employee-friend. The process of setting up a confrontation is demonstrated, including the pitfalls to successful preparation. Excellent for supplementing *The enablers* and for demonstrating enabling family dynamics, intervention, and teamwork. Also good for demonstrating how one can help the emissary from a troubled family motivate a chemically dependent person to seek treatment.

(33)
Audience   Health professionals

Further Information   American Hospital Association
                        Film Library
                        840 North Lake Shore Drive
                        Chicago, Illinois 60611

Resource: Film/videocassette

Cause the effect/Affect the cause. 1973; 23 min.; 16 mm or cassette; color.

Five hospital staff members and a police officer are confronted with an intoxicated patient. Each responds differently: each has a different effect on the patient's behavior. The film has three parts, each followed by questions pertaining to staff behavior and attitudes. Provocative, stimulating discussion about the history and proper medical and ethical management of this patient. Also good for presenting the attitudes toward an intoxicated person that can exist among hospital and law enforcement staff.

(34)
Audience   Physicians

Further Information   Office of Alcohol and Drug
                            Abuse Prevention
                          Health and Welfare Building
                          Hazen Drive
                          Concord, New Hampshire 03301

Resource: Videocassette alcoholism course

Alcoholism was produced for the physician either in private practice or in a hospital setting. It is most effective when presented to a small group of physicians. The package consists of video tapes, handouts, homework assignments, and a teacher's manual for the group leader. The material is organized into four 1-hour sessions:

> MODULE I introduces the system dynamics model and the twelve factors involved in chemical consumption. A case is presented early in the discussion and may be used by the participant to identify the factors discussed in the module.

> MODULE II introduces the physiological, social, and psychological factors involved in alcoholism and how they interact with each other.

> MODULE III introduces the concepts of the physiological addictive loops and emphasizes the factors related to tolerance and withdrawal.

> MODULE IV focuses on the treatment of the alcoholic. Using case studies from one's own practice, the participant analyzes the factors related to the patient's diagnosis and develops a rational treatment program based on information presented in the previous modules.

(35)
Audience   Health professionals

Further Information   Alcoholics Anonymous
                          Box 459
                          Grand Central Station
                          New York, New York 10163

Resource: Film/videocassette

Alcoholics anonymous: An inside view. 1979; 28 min.; 16 mm or video cassette.

An inside view of AA meetings from the smallest, intimate closed meetings to the large, open ones. It emphasizes the idea that AA is a way of life: any time two members get together there is an AA meeting.

Section Four: Examinations and Certification Procedures (36–38)

(36)

Audience	Medical school faculty
Further Information	Coordinator for Medical School Examination Services National Board of Medical Examiners 3930 Chestnut Street Philadelphia, Pennsylvania 19104 (215) 349-6400

Resource: Examination in drug and alcohol abuse

A Comprehensive Examination in Drug and Alcohol Abuse has been developed by a Task Force on Drug and Alcohol Abuse appointed by the National Board of Medical Examiners (NBME) and funded by the National Institute on Drug Abuse. This examination has been developed to assess student knowledge on substance abuse appropriate to the entire clinical portion of the medical school curriculum. The examination will be composed of approximately 120 items in multiple-choice format to be administered in a 2-hour time limit.

Participating schools will be provided total test percent correct scores for students, along with a mean percent correct score for a national sample of students. The NBME will not establish a pass/fail standard. Scores will be available approximately 2 weeks after the test materials are received by the NBME.

Examinations and corresponding keyword item analyses can be requested by submitting an NBME Subject Examination Services Order Form at least 5 weeks prior to the anticipated test administration date. Both this form and more detailed information about other National Board subject examinations and regulations governing their use may be obtained from the interested school's Executive Chief Proctor for National Board Examinations.

(37)
Audience   Physicians

Further Information   California Society for Treatment
                          of Alcoholism and Other Drug
                          Dependencies
                          Suite 1412
                          703 Market Street
                          San Francisco, California 94103
                          (415) 541-9286

Resource: Examination/certification

The California Society has developed a two-part examination. The first section consists of 100 multiple-choice questions; the second consists of Patient Management Problems, containing 100 items. The examination was administered in 1983 and 1984. One hundred eighty-three (183) physicians were certified by the Society. Certification indicates that a physician has demonstrated a degree of knowledge in the diagnosis and treatment of chemical dependence, commensurate with standards that identify a physician specialist as set forth by the California Society. Current plans call for future administrations of certifying examinations to be sponsored by the American Medical Society on Alcoholism and Other Drug Dependencies (see no. 38, below).

(38)
Audience   Physicians

Further Information   American Medical Society on Alcoholism
                          and Other Drug Dependencies
                          12 West 21st Street
                          New York, New York 10010
                          (212) 206-6770

Resource: Examination/certification

The American Medical Society on Alcoholism and Other Drug Dependencies (AMSAODD) plans to administer between December 1985 and February 1986 an examination similar in format to the California Society examination (see no. 37, above). Successful completion of the examination will make one eligible for certification by AMSAODD. The examination format and the significance of the certification will be similar to that now administered and granted by the California Society. With the initiation of the AMSOADD process, the Society's examinations and certification processes would be discontinued. The examination will be administered in several locales simultaneously. Courses in drugs and alcohol will be offered in the areas in which examinations are to be given.

Section Five: Organizations (39-45)

(39)

Audience   Medical educators

Further Information   (Individuals in this entry)

Resource: Career Teachers: Medical School Faculty in Drugs and Alcohol

In 1971, the National Institute on Drug Abuse and the National Institute on Alcohol Abuse and Alcoholism initiated a program to establish in U.S. medical schools a curriculum in drug abuse and alcoholism to educate medical students and physicians to properly prescribe licitly manufactured drugs. Faculty recipients of Career Teacher Grants are listed below.

Geary Alford, PhD
University of Mississippi
    Medical Center
Department of Psychiatry
2500 North State Street
Jackson, Mississippi 39216
(601) 968-3753

Rudy Arredondo, EdD
Texas Tech University
    School of Medicine
Department of Psychiatry
P.O. Box 4569
Lubbock, Texas 79409
(806) 743-2804

Mark Arthur, DMD
University of Maryland
    Dental School
Pharmacology Department
666 West Baltimore Street
Baltimore, Maryland 21201
(301) 528-7169

Roland M. Atkinson, MD
Health Science Center
University of Oregon
Veterans Administration
    Hospital
3710 S.W. Vets Hospital Road
Portland, Oregon 97201
(503) 222-9221, x 2500

Margaret Bean-Bayog, MD
Harvard Medical School
Cambridge Hospital
Cambridge, Massachusetts
  01246
(617) 734-9677

Joseph M. Benforado, MD
University of Wisconsin
1522 University Avenue
Madison, Wisconsin 53706
(608) 262-1923

Kenneth Blum, PhD
University of Texas
  Health Science Center
Department of Pharmacology
7703 Floyd Curl Drive
San Antonio, Texas 78284
(512) 691-6411

Louis Bozzetti, MD
Loma Linda University
  School of Medicine
Department of Psychiatry
Loma Linda, California 92354
(714) 825-7084, x 2205

Alan Brovar, MD
University of California at Los
  Angeles School of Medicine
941 Westwood Boulevard
Suite 205
Los Angeles, California 90024
(213) 208-5553

John N. Chappel, MD
University of Nevada
Behavioral Sciences
Anderson Health Science
  Building
Reno, Nevada 89507
(702) 784-4917

Don R. Cherek, PhD
Louisiana State University
  Medical Center
School of Medicine
Department of Psychiatry
P.O. Box 33932
Shreveport, Louisiana 71130
(318) 674-6040

Thomas J. Crowley, MD
University of Colorado
  Medical Center
Department of Psychiatry
4200 East Ninth Avenue
Denver, Colorado 80262
(303) 394-7573

Paul Cushman, MD
McGuire Veterans Administration Hospital
1201 Broadrock Road
Richmond, Virginia 23249
(804) 231-9011, x 206

Donald I. Davis, MD
Family Therapy Institute of
  Alexandria
220 South Washington Street
Alexandria, Virginia 22314
(703) 549-6001

John DiGregorio, MD, PhD
Hahnemann Medical College
Department of Pharmacology
235 North 15th Street
Philadelphia, Pennsylvania
  19102
(215) 448-8248

David Eiland, MD
University of Texas
Office of the Dean
Medical Branch
Administration Building
Galveston, Texas 77550
(713) 744-2528

Bradley D. Evans, MD
Philadelphia Veterans Administration Medical Center
DDTS – Building #7 (158)
University and Woodland Avenues
Philadelphia, Pennsylvania 19104
(215) 382-2400

John Femino, MD
Brown University
Roger Williams Hospital
825 Chalkstone Avenue
Providence, Rhode Island 02908
(401) 456-2362

William E. Flynn, MD
Georgetown University Hospital
Department of Psychiatry
Washington, D.C. 20007
(202) 625-7351

John E. Fryer, MD
Temple University
Department of Psychiatry
138 West Walnut Lane
Philadelphia, Pennsylvania 19144
(215) 848-2806

Marc Galanter, MD
Albert Einstein
College of Medicine
Department of Psychiatry
Bronx, New York 10461
(212) 430-5522, x 5526

Donald M. Gallant, MD
Tulane Medical Center
Department of Psychiatry
1415 Tulane Avenue
New Orleans, Louisiana 70112
(504) 588-5405

Peter Gessner, PhD
State University of New York-Buffalo
Department of Pharmacology
122 Farber Hall
Buffalo, New York 14214
(716) 831-3295

Jules Golden, MD
University of Utah
College of Medicine
Veterans Administration
Medical Center (116A)
Salt Lake City, Utah 84148

John Griffin, MD
Emory University
Department of Psychiatry
Georgia Mental Health Institute
1256 Briarcliff Road, N.E.
Room 166A
Atlanta, Georgia 30306
(404) 894-5869

Alyce C. Gullattee, MD
Howard University
Department of Psychiatry
520 "W" Street, N.W.
Washington, D.C. 20059
(202) 745-6689

James Halikas, MD
Medical College of Wisconsin
Division of Alcohol and
  Chemical Dependency
Department of Psychiatry
9191 Watertown Plank Road
Milwaukee, Wisconsin 53226
(414) 257-7011

Harlan Hill, PhD
c/o Fred Hutchinson Cancer
  Research Center
Room 122
1124 Columbia Street
Seattle, Washington 98104
(206) 467-4587

Andrew K. S. Ho, PhD
University of Illinois
Peoria School of Medicine
Division of Pharmacology
123 S.W. Glendale
Peoria, Illinois 61605
(309) 671-3122

Jeptha Hostetler, PhD
Ohio State University
Department of Preventive
  Medicine
320 W. 10th Avenue
Room 216-B
Columbus, Ohio 43210
(614) 421-3925

George Jackson, MD
Duke University Medical
  Center
Box 2914
Durham, North Carolina
  27710
(919) 684-3225

Kim A. Keeley, MD
117 State Street
Brooklyn, New York 11201
(212) 624-8599

Ronald S. Krug, PhD
2401 Old Farm Road
Edmond, Oklahoma 73034
(405) 341-6862

Leon Kuhs, MD
Northwestern University
  Medical School
Department of Psychiatry
Institute of Psychiatry
320 East Huron
Chicago, Illinois 60611
(312) 263-5362

Robert Landeen, MD
Department of Psychiatry
Room TF 104
Stanford Medical Center
Stanford, California 94305
(415) 497-6661

Joseph Levin, EdD
University of Illinois
School of Public Health
P.O. Box 6998-SPH 321
Chicago, Illinois 60680
(312) 996-6385

Jerome Levy, PhD
University of New Mexico
School of Medicine
Department of Psychiatry
930 Stanford, N.E.
Albuquerque, New Mexico
 87110
(505) 242-4442

Michael Liepman, MD
Veterans Administration
 Medical Center (116A6)
Davis Park
Providence, Rhode Island
 02908
(401) 273-7100, x 481

James Lukes, PhD
University of Massachusetts
Medical Center
Department of Family and
 Community Medicine
55 Lake Avenue North
Worcester, Massachusetts
 01605
(617) 856-3021

Karen Mack, MD
Cheshire Hospital
Department of Psychiatry
Keene, New Hampshire 03431
(603) 352-4111

Marvin Mathews, MD
University of Hawaii
Department of Psychiatry
Leahi Hospital
3675 Kilauea Avenue
Honolulu, Hawaii 96816
(808) 732-6658

Robert Millman, MD
Cornell University Medical
 College
411 East 69th Street
New York, New York 10021
(212) 472-5243

John Morgan, MD
The City College of the City of
 New York
Sophie Davis Center for
 Biomedical Education
138th Street and Convent
 Avenue
New York, New York 10031
(212) 690-8255

E. Don Nelson, PharmD
University of Cincinnati
DPIC-7702 Bridge
Medical Science Building
231 Bethesda Avenue
Cincinnati, Ohio 45267
(513) 872-4066

Robert Niven, MD
Director
National Institute on Alcohol
 Abuse and Alcoholism
5600 Fishers Lane,
 Room 16-105
Rockville, Maryland 20857
(301) 443-3885

James O'Brien, MD, PhD
University of Connecticut
School of Medicine
Department of Psychiatry
Farmington, Connecticut
 06032
(203) 674-3422

Paul Pascarosa, MD
Pulaski Community Hospital
P.O. Box 759
Pulaski, Virginia 24301
(703) 980-6822

Robert J. Rhodes, PhD
3608 West 84th Street
Shawnee Mission, Kansas
 66206
(913) 649-4171

Jack M. Rogers, MD
Bowman Gray School of
 Medicine
Department of Psychiatry
Hawthorne Road
Winston Salem,
 North Carolina 27103
(919) 748-3608

Henry L. Rosett, MD
Boston University
Department of Psychiatry
561 Barnstable Road
West Newton, Massachusetts
 02165
(617) 527-0577

Kenneth S. Russell, EdD
CHEP Coordinator
Cooperative Health Education
 Program
VAMROC 11C
Togus, Maine 04330
(207) 623-8411, x 513

Gene Sausser, PhD
University of South Carolina
 School of Medicine
Department of Neuropsychiatry
 and Behavioral Science
P.O. Box 119
Columbia, South Carolina
 29202
(803) 758-8645

Sidney Schnoll, MD, PhD
Northwestern University
Division of Substance Abuse
Institute of Psychiatry
320 East Huron
Chicago, Illinois 60611
(312) 936-1194

Eugene P. Schoener, PhD
Wayne State University
School of Medicine
Department of Pharmacology
540 East Canfield
Detroit, Michigan 48201
(313) 577-1570

John Severinghaus, MD
Veterans Administration
 Hospital
Alcoholism and Rehabilitation
 Program
White River Junction,
 Vermont 05001
(802) 295-9363, x 451

Douglas Soule, PhD
University of South Dakota
School of Medicine
Department of Psychiatry
2501 West 22
Sioux Falls, South Dakota
 57105
(605) 339-6785

Claudio Toro, MD
Psychiatry Associates, P.A.
P.O. Box 2992
Birmingham, Alabama 35212
(205) 838-1203

George S. Tyner, MD
Texas Tech University
Department of Ophthalmology
Health Sciences Center
3601 4th Street
Suite 3A-124
Lubbock, Texas 79424
(806) 743-2381

Lucas S. Van Orden, MD, PhD
Rural Route 2
Iowa City, Iowa 52240
(319) 351-8038

Alan Wartenberg, MD
Medical College of Wisconsin
Department of Medicine
8700 West Wisconsin Avenue
P.O. Box 189
Milwaukee, Wisconsin 53226
(414) 257-5787

Richard L. Weddige, MD
Texas Tech University
School of Medicine
Department of Psychiatry
P.O. Box 4569
Lubbock, Texas 79409
(806) 743-2800

Joseph Westermeyer, MD, PhD
University of Minnesota
Department of Psychiatry
University of Minnesota Hospitals
Box 393 Mayo
Minneapolis, Minnesota 55455
(612) 373-8102

Jocelyn Whiten, PhD
Charles R. Drew Medical School Department of Community Medicine
12021 South Wilmington Avenue
Los Angeles, California 90059
(213) 603-8166

Charles L. Whitfield, MD
University of Maryland School of Medicine
721 West Redwood Street
Baltimore, Maryland 21201
(301) 528-6800

Ken Williams, MD
Neumann Center for Addiction Treatment
St. Joseph's Hospital
12th and Walnut Streets
Reading, Pennsylvania 19603
(215) 378-2180

CAREER TEACHER TRAINING CENTERS FACULTIES

DOWNSTATE MEDICAL CENTER

Charles Buchwald, PhD
858 East 23rd Street
Brooklyn, New York 11210
(212) 951-7724

Benjamin Kissin, MD
525 East 86th Street
New York, New York 10028

Joel Solomon, MD
300 West End Avenue
New York, New York 10023
(212) 595-9119

BAYLOR COLLEGE OF MEDICINE

Alex Pokorny, MD
Department of Psychiatry
Baylor College of Medicine
1200 Moursund Avenue
Houston, Texas 77030
(713) 799-4865

Joseph Schoolar, MD, PhD
Department of Psychiatry
Baylor College of Medicine
1200 Moursund Avenue
Houston, Texas 77030
(713) 799-4865

(40)

Audience Medical educators

Further Information David C. Lewis, MD
President
Association for Medical Education and
 Research in Substance Abuse
Box G
Brown University
Providence, Rhode Island 02912
(401) 863-3172

Resource: Professional association

The Association for Medical Education and Research in Substance Abuse (AMERSA) meets annually in November to discuss research and clinical findings in drugs of abuse and alcohol, and their implications for medical education. Members are medical educators from approximately 80 U.S. medical schools. Membership is open to all physicians, medical school faculty, and health professions educators.

(41)
Audience   Medical educators
                   Health professions educators

Further Information   (Individuals in this entry)

Resource: Health professions educators in drugs and alcohol

A Health Professions Task Force was formed in 1974 and again in 1978 to develop education resources and programs for physicians, osteopaths, nurses, psychologists, pharmacists, physicians' assistants, and social workers. Representatives of these professions as well as medical librarians, health educators, and government drug and alcohol institutes' representatives were members of the Task Force.

The Task Force's Committee on Licensure and Certification worked with six medical specialty licensing boards and with the Nurse, Osteopath, Psychology, Social Work, Physician Assistant, and Pharmacy Boards to develop drug and alcohol questions for certifying and licensing examinations. The Committee on Professional Education conducted and published surveys on drug and alcohol education in the professional schools and worked with representatives of each of the national professional associations to develop education materials and programs for the professions.

The Task Force is no longer active as a group. The names of the members are given below, since each is knowledgeable about drug and alcohol education in his or her field.

Rita Albery, RN, MS
NIAAA
5600 Fishers Lane
Parklawn Building, Room 16C10
Rockville, Maryland 20857
(301) 443-3860
(Nurse)

Jane Bemko, MLS
Alcoholism Treatment Center
Texas Research Institute for
    Mental Sciences
1300 Moursund
Houston, Texas 77030
(713) 797-6346
(Medical Librarian)

Charles Buchwald, PhD
Career Teacher Center
Downstate Medical Center
450 Clarkson Avenue – Box 129
Brooklyn, New York 11203
(212) 270-3150
(Psychologist)

James Callahan, DPA
Division of Cancer Prevention
    and Control
National Cancer Institute
National Institutes of Health
Building 31, Room 11A–19
9000 Rockville Pike

Bethesda, Maryland 20205
(301) 496-1071
(Medical/Health Professions Educator)

Annie J. Carter, RN, EdD
Meharry Medical College
Department of Nursing Education
Nashville, Tennessee 37208
(615) 327-6497
(Nurse)

Eileen Corrigan, DSW
Rutgers State University
Graduate School of Social Work
CN5058
New Brunswick, New Jersey 08903
(210) 932-7194
(Social Worker)

Joseph V. Fisher, MD
Department of Family Practice
College of Medicine
Medical University of South Carolina
80 Boise Street
Charleston, South Carolina 29401
(803) 792-2411
(Physician – Family Practice)

John B. Griffin, Jr., MD
Emory University
School of Medicine
Georgia Mental Health Institute
1256 Briarcliff Road, N.E., Room 166A
Atlanta, Georgia 30306
(404) 894-5869
(Physician – Child Psychiatrist)

Edith Heinemann, MA, FAAN
Alcoholism Nursing Program, SC-78
Department of Psychosocial Nursing
School of Nursing
University of Washington
Seattle, Washington 98195
(206) 543-6065
(Nurse)

Nancy Humphreys, DSW
Michigan State University
School of Social Work
254 Baker Hall
E. Lansing, Michigan 48824
(517) 355-7515
(Social Worker)

Norman P. Johnson, PhD
Physicians' Assistants Program
Western Michigan University
Kalamazoo, Michigan 49008
(616) 383-6118
(Physician Assistant Educator)

Brian Katcher, PharmD
1927 Page Street
San Francisco, California 94117
(415) 386-5524
(Pharmacist)

Claire Lyons-Callahan, MA
1213 Fallsmead Way
Potomac, Maryland 20854
(301) 340-2291
(Health Professions Educator)

E. Don Nelson, PharmD
University of Cincinnati
DPIC – 7702 Bridge

Medical Science Building
231 Bethesda Avenue
Cincinnati, Ohio 45267
(513) 872-4066
(Pharmacist)

Sidney A. Orgel, PhD
State University of New York
Upstate Medical Center
Department of Psychiatry
750 East Adams Street
Syracuse, New York 13210
(315) 473-5630
(Psychologist)

Al Rosen, DO
321 Northlake Boulevard
Suite 101
North Palm Beach, Florida 33408
(305) 844-2161
(Osteopath)

Sidney Schnoll, MD, PhD
Northwestern University
Division of Substance Abuse
Institute of Psychiatry
320 East Huron
Chicago, Illinois 60611
(312) 649-8713
(Physician, Pharmacologist)

Bernard Sobel, DO
Valley Forge Medical Center
1033 Germantown Pike
Norristown, Pennsylvania 19403
(215) 539-8500
(Osteopath)

Joel Solomon, MD
300 West End Avenue
New York, New York 10023
(212) 595-9119
(Physician, Psychiatrist)

(42)

Audience Health professionals

Further Information National Clearinghouse for Alcohol Information
P.O. Box 2345
Rockville, Maryland 20852
(301) 468-2600

Resource: Clearinghouse

The clearinghouse is an information service of the National Institute on Alcohol Abuse and Alcoholism (NIAAA). Information is gathered from worldwide sources and made available to members of the professions and the public through several publications and services.

(43)

Audience Health professionals

Further Information   National Clearinghouse on Drug Abuse
Information
P.O. Box 416
Kensington, Maryland 20795
(301) 443-6500

Resource: Clearinghouse

The clearinghouse is an information service of the National Institute on Drug Abuse (NIDA). Information is gathered from worldwide sources and made available to members of the professions and the public through several publications and services. A publications list is available on request.

(44)
Audience   Health professionals

Further Information   Addiction Research Foundation
33 Russell Street
Toronto, Ontario M5S 2S1
(807) 595-6000

Resource: (See no. 26, above)

(45)
Audience   Health professionals

Further Information   Center of Alcohol Studies
Research Information and Publications Division
Rutgers University
P.O. Box 969
Piscataway, New Jersey 08854
(201) 932-3510

Resource: Literature abstracts

The Research Information and Publications Division of the Center of Alcohol Studies collects, classifies, and abstracts scientific literature on alcohol and alcoholism. This organized knowledge is available through several publications and services.

PART II:

PRESCRIBING, DISPENSING, AND ADMINISTERING CONTROLLED SUBSTANCES

Section One: General Texts and Resources (46–58)

(46)

Audience Physicians
Health professionals

Further Information American Medical Association
Order Department
P.O. Box 10946
Chicago, Illinois 60610

Resource: Book

AMA drug evaluations (5th ed.). Chicago, Illinois: American Medical Association, 1983.

The *AMA-DE* gives physicians and other health care professionals up-to-date information on the clinical use of drugs most commonly prescribed or administered by physicians in the United States. The eighty-four chapters were written by professional staff of the AMA's Division of Drugs, and reviewed by more than 500 consultants and medical staffs of the pharmaceutical manufacturers and by designees or members of the American Society for Clinical Pharmacology and Therapeutics. The first three chapters contain general information on prescribing practices and regulatory agencies, drug interactions and adverse drug reactions, drug response variation, and dosage information. In the remaining chapters, drugs within a therapeutic category are reviewed in the chapter introduction. This is followed by evaluations of individual drugs: actions and uses; pharmacokinetics, adverse reactions and precautions; and routes, usual dosage, and preparations. References.

(47)

Audience Physicians
Pharmacists
Registered nurses

	Clinical and administrative support personnel
Further Information	GTE Telenet Medical Information Network
12490 Sunrise Valley Drive
Reston, Virginia 22096
(703) 442-2500
(800) 368-4215

Resource: Computerized clinical data bases

The AMA and GTE have developed computer data bases on "Drug Information," "Disease Information," "Medical Procedure Coding and Nomenclature," "Socio/Economic Bibliographic Information," "Clinical Literature," "Continuing Education," and the AMA-NET Medical News Service of daily popular press medical news from several specialty areas. An Electronic Mail Service is also available for communicating within the medical community.

(48)

Audience	Clinical pharmacists
Physicians
Nurse practitioners
Physicians' assistants
Further Information	Applied Therapeutics, Inc.
P.O. Box 31-747
San Francisco, California 94131

Resource: Book

Katcher, B. S., Young, L., and Koda-Kimble, M.A. *Applied therapeutics: The clinical use of drugs.* San Francisco: Applied Therapeutics, 1983.

The book illustrates the appropriate clinical application of pharmacology and pharmacokinetics to specific patient problems. This is done through the use of case histories, questions, and referenced responses to bring into focus the nature of the decision-making process. References.

(49)

Audience	Prescribers
Further Information	(Publisher)

Resource: Reference book

Physician's desk reference (37th ed.). Oradell, New Jersey: Medical Economics Company, Inc., 1983.

Under the Federal Food, Drug, and Cosmetic Act, a drug approved for marketing may be labeled, promoted, and advertised by the manufacturer only for those uses for which the drug's safety and effectiveness have been established and which the FDA has approved. The Code of Federal Regulations 201.100(d)(i) pertaining to labeling for prescription products requires that for the *Physician's desk reference* (PDR) content, "indications and usage, dosages, routes, methods, and frequency and duration of administration, description, clinical pharmacology and supply and any relevant warnings, hazards, contradiction, adverse reactions, potential for drug abuse and dependence, overdosage and precautions," must be the "same in language and emphasis" as the approved labeling for the product. For products that do not have official package circulars, the publisher has emphasized to manufacturers the necessity of describing such products comprehensively so that physicians would have access to all information essential for intelligent and informed prescribing. In organizing and presenting the material in the PDR, the publisher is providing all the information made available to PDR by manufacturers (Publisher).

(50)

Audience	Physicians
Further Information	The Haworth Press, Inc. 28 East 22nd Street New York, New York 10010

Resource: Prescribing monograph

Cohen, S., Buchwald, C., Solomon, J., Callahan, J., and Katz, D. (Eds.) *Frequently prescribed and abused drugs: Their indications, efficacy and rational prescribing.* New York: The Haworth Press, 1982.

The monograph has six chapters. The first, "Drug Abuse and the Prescribing Physician" (Cohen), discusses diversion, the need for sensitivity to the problem of drug abuse in prescribing psychotropic drugs, and the physician-patient-prescribing relationship. The other chapters address "Psychotropic Drug Interactions" (Hollister), "Anxiety: Its Meaning and Psychotropic Drug Treatment" (Wesson), "The Prescription of Stimulants and Anorectics" (Smith and Seymour), "Pain"

(Schnoll), and "The Prescription of Hypnotic Drugs" (Kales, Kales, and Scharf). The monograph contains Pre- and Post-Tests.

(51)
Audience   Physicians

Further Information   American Medical Association
                        Order Department
                        P.O. Box 10946
                        Chicago, Illinois 60610

Resource: Chapter

Wilford, B. B. Prescribing practices and drug abuse, Chapter 10. IN: *Drug abuse: A guide for the primary care physician.* Chicago, Illinois: American Medical Association, 1981.

The chapter discusses underprescribing and overprescribing; summarizes the "Guidelines for Prescribers of Controlled Substances" developed by DEA in collaboration with other professional organizations and federal agencies; summarizes the five Schedules established by the Controlled Substances Act; discusses the indications for prescribing psychoactive drugs and their abuse potential; and addresses the issues of improving patient compliance, identifying the "patient hustler," and developing a rational approach to prescribing. References.

(52)
Audience   Physicians

Further Information   California Medical Association
                        Task Force on Prescription Drug Abuse
                        44 Gough Street
                        San Francisco, California 94103
                        (415) 863-5522, x 403

Resource: Videocassette

Guidelines for prescribing any dependence-producing drug. 40 minutes; 3/4" videocassette; color.

This is a videotape of a lecture outlining five principles to be followed in issuing a prescription for any dependence-producing drug: diagnosis, dosage, duration, dependence, and discontinuance.

(53)
Audience	Physicians
	Pharmacists
Further Information	Dr. J. Stephen Kennedy
	Project Sleep
	9C-09
	5600 Fishers Lane
	Rockville, Maryland 20857
	(301) 443-3948

Resource: Sleep disorder program

Information from the Sleep Disorder Program includes a description of Project Sleep, a list of sleep disorder centers, and information on sleep disorder treatment.

(54)
Audience	Physicians
	Pharmacists
Further Information	Medical School Libraries
	or
	Director
	Medical Science Liaison Program
	Upjohn Pharmaceuticals
	Unit 92-79-243
	Kalamazoo, Michigan 49001
	(616) 323-6008

Resource: Slides and audiocassettes

This is an educational package developed by the sleep treatment research community that includes slides, audiocassettes, and printed materials in six 1-hour lecture modules.

(55)
Audience	Physicians
	Pharmacists
Further Information	National Academy of Sciences Press
	2101 Constitution Avenue, N.W.
	Washington, D.C. 20418
	(202) 334-2000

Resource: Report

Sleeping pills, insomnia and medical practice. Washington, D.C.: National Academy of Sciences, 1979.

The report contains chapters on epidemiology of sleep complaints and prescribing practices, public health problems associated with hypnotic use, research on insomnia, and an assessment of the hazards and benefits of hypnotic drugs.

(56)

Audience	Physicians
Further Information	California Medical Association Task Force on Prescription Drug Abuse 44 Gough Street San Francisco, California 94103 (415) 863-5522, ext. 403

Resource: Videocassette

Prescribing for insomnia and anxiety. 40 min.; 3/4" videocassette; color.

The videocassette portrays role play prescribing by "Dr. Naive," "Dr. Quick-to-Conclude," and "Dr. Scientific." A physician commentator interprets the behaviors and how they may lead to prescription drug abuse or failure to respond to the patient's problem. He describes principles for prescribing for insomnia. Another physician commentator analyzes whether the prescribing pattern is within community standards from the viewpoint of the Board of Medical Quality Assurance's Medical Consultant, or plaintiff's attorney.

(57)

Audience	Physicians
Further Information	Local DuPont pharmaceutical representative

Resource: Self-study course: videocassettes/study guides

Practical concepts on the management of pain. 15 min.; videocassette; color.
Treating acute pain effectively. 15 min.; videocassette; color.
Post-operative pain management: A discussion with John Bonica. 15 min.; videocassette; color.

Individualizing cancer pain management. 15 min.; videocassette; color.

The study guides for the pain management self-study course contain summaries of the video presentation, an application section, a self-assessment quiz and answers, and a bibliography. A moderator's booklet is available for each unit. The program is sponsored by the University of Washington School of Medicine. Continuing Education Units are available.

(58)
Audience	Health professionals
Further Information	Order Section, GSA
	National Archives and Record Service
	Washington, DC 20409
	(301) 763-1896

Resource: Film/videocassette

Elder ed. 1977; 30 min.; 16 mm or cassette; color.

Elder ed is a three-part film on the problems associated with prescription drugs and the elderly. The first part describes the "new world" of drugs, which is confusing to some elderly persons. The second part portrays buying drugs wisely and includes a discussion with pharmacists regarding generic versus brand names. The final segment outlines ways to keep track of how the drugs are being taken (compliance).

Section Two: Diversion for Purposes of Abuse (59–68)

(59)
Audience	Prescribers
	Dispensers
	Manufacturers
	Regulators
	Law enforcement personnel
Further Information	Administrator
	Substance Abuse Unit
	Health and Human Behavior Program

American Medical Association
535 N. Dearborn Street
Chicago, Illinois 60610

Resource: Informal steering committee on prescription drug abuse

In November 1981, the AMA formed the Informal Steering Committee on Prescription Drug Abuse with twenty organizations representing prescribers, dispensers, manufacturers, regulators, and enforcement agencies. The committee has the following objectives: (1) arrive at agreements on the nature of the problem and what to do about it; (2) support interdisciplinary conferences to initiate understanding of the problems and solutions at state levels; (3) urge the formation in each state of an interdisciplinary task force to coordinate problem identification, resource identification, goal setting, and action; (4) establish a financial clearinghouse to match the resource needs of state program planners with available sources of support; (5) endorse the development of methods of longitudinal instruction in prescribing; (6) develop a data analysis model (PADS: Prescription Abuse Data Synthesis) to identify sources of diversion; (7) study legislative issues that affect regulation, enforcement, and intervention with prescribers and dispensers; (8) draft model legislation, as needed; (9) explore the feasibility of a national clearinghouse to exchange information among state authorities about disciplinary actions against prescribers; (10) study the effects of multiple-copy prescription systems on diversion and the quality of patient care; and (11) improve the ability of physicians to diagnose and treat patients dependent on drugs and alcohol. (Skom, J. An interprofessional view of the problem of prescription drug abuse. *Pharmacy Times*, May 1983, 70–74.)

(60)

Audience   Physicians

Further Information   Manager
Scientific and Public Information
Roche Laboratories
Division of Hoffmann-La Roche, Inc.
Nutley, New Jersey 07110
(201) 235-3510

Resource: Public service message

The *Medical director's page* is a series of public service messages on "Recognizing the Manipulative Patient," "Protecting Your Prescription," "The Fraudulent Prescription," "The Prudent Use of Psychotherapeutic Agents," "National Patterns of Psychoactive Drug Use," "Noncompliance," "Psychoactive Drugs and the Controlled Substance Act," and "The Family Physician and the Problem Drinker."

(61)

Audience   Prescribers of controlled substances

Further Information   Voluntary Compliance Coordinator
Drug Enforcement Administration
1405 I Street, N.W.
Washington, D.C. 20537
(202) 633-1091

Resource: Guidelines

Guidelines for prescribers of controlled substances. Washington, D.C.: Drug Enforcement Administration, 1980.

These guidelines provide and establish acceptable professional responses to the demands of the Controlled Substances Act. They provide a common sense approach to encourage voluntary compliance by the prescribing professions. They were prepared under the auspices of the DEA/Practitioners Working Committee and approved by the American Dental Association, American Medical Association, American Nurses Association, American Osteopathic Association, American Podiatry Association, American Veterinary Medicine Association, the National Institute on Drug Abuse, and the Drug Enforcement Administration.

(62)

Audience   Physicians

Further Information   Drug Enforcement Administration
Office of Public Affairs
1405 I Street, N.W.
Washington, D.C. 20537
(202) 633-1249

Resource: Booklet

Physician's manual: An informational outline of the Controlled Substances Act of 1970. Washington, D.C.: Drug Enforcement Administration, 1978.

This booklet was prepared by the Office of Compliance and Regulatory Affairs as part of DEA's Voluntary Compliance Program to assist physicians in their understanding of the Controlled Substances Act of 1970 and its implementing regulations as they pertain to medical practitioners. The booklet has been reviewed and endorsed by the American Dental Association, American Medical Association, American Nurses Association, American Osteopathic Association, American Podiatry Association, and American Veterinary Medicine Association.

(63)

Audience	Physicians
	Osteopaths
Further Information	Division of Medical Education
	American Medical Association
	535 N. Dearborn Street
	Chicago, Illinois 60610
	(312) 645-4639

Resource: Videocassette, workbook, and instructor's guide

Prescribing psychoactive drugs: How does your practice measure up? 1985; 43 min.; cassette or 16 mm; color.

The general purposes of this continuing medical education program developed by the AMA and Haight-Ashbury Training and Education Projects are to teach physicians to recognize deceptive, drug-seeking behavior and to respond appropriately. The goal is to improve patient care and public health by minimizing the opportunities for diversion or illicit use of controlled drugs. The second, but equally important, goal is to emphasize to physicians the potential consequences to them of misprescribing, even if the misprescribing is the result of deception or theft.

The program is in three parts: a 43-minute video, a workbook or resource guide, and an instructor's guide. The workbook goes into detail regarding controlled drugs and drug diversion, including pharmacology, indications and contradictions, medico-legal aspects, and identification and referral of drug-dependent patients. The instructor's guide provides the local instructor with the tools to generate discussion, elaborate on points made in the video, and apply the video to local laws and practices.

(64)
Audience   Physicians

Further Information   Drug Enforcement Administration
Office of Public Affairs
1405 I Street, N.W.
Washington, D.C. 20537
(202) 633-1249

Resource: Booklet

Don't be deceived by a drug addict. Washington, D.C.: Drug Enforcement Administration, 1976.
    A true narration by a drug addict of ways in which he deceived doctors and obtained prescriptions. (Reprinted by DEA from *AMA News*, November 22, 1976, *19*, 46, 1–4).

(65)
Audience   Pharmacists

Further Information   Drug Enforcement Administration
Office of Public Affairs
1405 I Street, N.W.
Washington, D.C. 20537
(202) 633-1249

Resource: Booklet

Pharmacist's manual: An informational outline of the Controlled Substances Act of 1970. Washington, D.C.: Drug Enforcement Administration, 1980.
    This booklet was prepared by the Office of Compliance and Regulatory Affairs as part of DEA's Voluntary Compliance Program to assist pharmacists in their understanding of the Controlled Substances Act of 1970 and its implementing regulations.

(66)
Audience   Physicians

Further Information   California Medical Association

Task Force on Prescription Drug Abuse
44 Gough Street
San Francisco, California 94103
(415) 863-5522, ext. 403

Resource: Videocassette

Games patients play. 40 min.; 3/4" videocassette; color.

Role players portray the manipulative patient, the sexually seductive patient, the sophisticated aggressive patient, and the patient who pleads. Physician commentators discuss how physicians can distinguish the knowing from the unknowing manipulators and how he/she can counteract the manipulation.

(67)

Audience	Pharmacists
Further Information	National Association of Boards of Pharmacy Foundation One East Wacker Drive Suite 2210 Chicago, Illinois 60601 (312) 467-6220

Resource: Videocassettes/study guides

Professional and legal responsibilities in pharmacy practice: The Federal Food, Drug, and Cosmetic Act. 48 min.; videocassette.

Professional and legal responsibilities in pharmacy practice: The Controlled Substance Act. 67 min.; videocassette.

The videocassettes and study guides discuss the historical development of the Acts and present scenarios of how they apply in the practice of pharmacy. The programs should be accompanied by a live presentation by a representative of the local state board of pharmacy to discuss state and federal laws in relation to the videocassettes. Pre- and Post-Knowledge Evaluations are included. Continuing Education Units are available through the National Association of Boards of Pharmacy (NABP) and the NABP Foundation.

(68)

Audience Professional association directors
Licensing board directors
Professional school deans

Further Information   Voluntary Compliance Coordinator
Drug Enforcement Administration
1405 I Street, N.W.
Washington, D.C. 20537
(202) 633-1091

Resource: Newsletter

Registrant facts. Washington, D.C.: Drug Enforcement Administration.

Registrant facts is published biannually. Volume 9, No. 1, 1983 has articles on "Stress Clinics," "Impaired Physicians and Prescribing Practices," "Hospital Security," and "The Role of the State Medical Board in Curtailing Diversion."

Section Three: The Impaired Professional (69–78)

(69)
Audience   Physicians

Further Information   Health and Human Behavior Program
American Medical Association
535 N. Dearborn Street
Chicago, Illinois 60610

Resource: Newsletter

The AMA impaired physician newsletter. Chicago, Illinois: American Medical Association.

The newsletter is published quarterly and contains information on public and private programs for impaired physicians. Statistics on impairment are published as available.

(70)
Audience   Physicians

Further Information   (1975, 1977, and 1978)
Health and Human Behavior Program
American Medical Association
535 N. Dearborn Street
Chicago, Illinois 60610

(1980)
Order Department OP-129
American Medical Association
P.O. Box 10946
Chicago, Illinois 60610

Resource: Conference proceedings

Steindler, E. M. *The impaired physician: An interpretive summary of the AMA conference on "The Disabled Doctor: Challenge to the Profession,"* April 11–12, 1975, San Francisco.

Hugunen, M. B. (Ed.). *Helping the impaired physician: Proceedings of the AMA conference on "The Impaired Physician: Answering the Challenge,"* February 4–6, 1977, Atlanta.

Robertson, J. J. (Ed.). *The impaired physician: Proceedings of the third AMA conference on "The Impaired Physician,"* September 29–October 1, 1978, Minneapolis.

Robertson, J. J. (Ed.). *The impaired physician: Building well-being: Proceedings of the fourth AMA conference on "The Impaired Physician,"* October 30–November 1, 1980, Baltimore.

(71)
Audience	Physicians
Further Information	Order Department OP-083 American Medical Association P.O. Box 10946 Chicago, Illinois 60610

Resource: Book

Tobarz, J. P., Bremer, W., and Peters, K. *Beyond survival.* Chicago, Illinois: American Medical Association, 1979.

The authors discuss the scope and nature of impairment among residents and physicians in general, offer a model program for helping the impaired resident, provide guidelines for establishing a program, and discuss the concept of well-being and approaches to achieving it. References and annotated bibliography.

(72)
Audience	Physicians Medical students

Further Information Biomedical Communications
Tulane Medical School
1430 Tulane Avenue
New Orleans, Louisiana 70117

Resource: Videocassette

Alcohol and drug abuse among physicians. 1979; 52 min.; videocassette; color.

Candid interviews with two rehabilitated doctors and their wives about their personal experience with alcohol and drugs. The interviews were conducted, unrehearsed, before an audience of 260 freshmen medical students at Tulane.

(73)
Audience Pharmacists

Further Information American Pharmaceutical Association
2215 Constitution Avenue, N.W.
Washington, D.C. 20037
(202) 429-7561

Resource: Course (Summer)

The American Pharmaceutical Association and the University of Utah cosponsor courses for those who deal with pharmacists and students who are dependent on alcohol or other drugs. Members of state pharmaceutical association committees, state board of pharmacy officials, pharmacy managers, pharmacy school representatives, and pharmacy students are invited. Participants are given assistance in developing and applying guidelines for the operation of referral, treatment, and rehabilitation programs. Continuing Education Units are available through the University of Utah College of Pharmacy.

(74)
Audience Pharmacists

Further Information American Pharmaceutical Association
2215 Constitution Avenue, N.W.
Washington, D.C. 20037
(202) 429-7532

Resource: Guidelines

Guidelines for planning and implementing programs for impaired pharmacists. Washington, D.C.: American Pharmaceutical Association, 1980.

(75)
Audience   Nurses

Further Information   (See below.)

Resource: Impaired practice resources

Several sources have information on impaired nurse programs. Among them are the following:

1. *Programs:* Information on impaired practice programs may be obtained from the individual State Nurses Association or from:
         The American Nurses Association
         2420 Pershing Road
         Kansas City, Missouri 64108
         (816) 474-5720

2. *Brochure: Addictions and psychological dysfunctions: The profession's response to the problem.* Kansas City, Missouri: American Nurses Association.

3. *Brochure:* A pamphlet for administrators regarding impaired practice is available from:
         Florida Nurses Association
         P.O. Box 6985
         Orlando, Florida 32853
         (305) 896-3261

4. *Organizations:* Drugs and Alcohol Nurses Association (DANA)
         P.O. Box 371
         College Park, Maryland 20740

         National Nurses' Society on Addictions
         6005 Mastway
         Suite 100
         Shawnee Mission, Kansas 66202

(76)
Audience   Nurses

Further Information   Project Director
                                  Nurses Assisting Nurses

College of Nursing
University of Kentucky
Lexington, Kentucky 40536 0232
(606) 233-5406

Resource: Impaired practice program

Nurses Assisting Nurses is (1) a counseling service for registered nurses whose practice is compromised due to substance abuse and/or emotional stress, (2) a research project to explore professional nursing issues as they relate to the problem of impairment, and (3) an educational program that provides information regarding this issue.

(77)

Audience	Dentists
Further Information	Secretary
	Council on Dental Practice
	American Dental Association
	211 East Chicago Avenue
	Chicago, Illinois 60611
	(312) 440-2750

Resource: Clearinghouse

The American Dental Association's (ADA) Council on Dental Practice serves as a clearinghouse and national source of information on alcohol and chemical dependency programs for the dental profession. The ADA publishes a list of these programs and has information on state dental practice acts and a model impaired dentist act.

(78)

Audience	Physicians
	Veterinarians
	Osteopaths
	Podiatrists
	Pharmacists
	Dentists
	Nurses
Further Information	Director
	Impaired Health Professionals Program
	3995 South Cobb Drive

Smyrna, Georgia 30080
(404) 434-4567

Resource: Impaired professionals treatment program

The Disabled Doctors Program was founded in 1975 by the Medical Association of Georgia for the treatment of chemically impaired or emotionally disturbed doctors. The program has evolved into the Impaired Health Professionals Program, which includes the treatment of chemically dependent nurses, pharmacists, and dentists. All programs bear the support of their respective societies.

The program has four phases of treatment. In the first phase, the patient is detoxified and participates in an intense 29-day program on an inpatient basis. During the second month of treatment, the patient moves to a residential treatment facility where he or she is treated on an outpatient basis. The impaired health professional participates in the treatment of others suffering from diseases similar to his or her own during the third phase. In the final phase, the health professional returns to his or her practice or place of employment and is closely monitored for 20 months.

Section Four: State-wide Programs (79–91)

(79)
Audience   Health professions

Further Information Committee on Prescription Drug Misuse
Division of Substance Abuse Services
Two World Trade Center
67th Floor
New York, New York 10047
(212) 488-4253

Resource: State-wide committee

The Committee on Prescription Drug Misuse was established by the New York State Division of Substance Abuse Services in 1978. The Committee, composed of volunteer experts in the fields of medicine, industry, labor, pharmaceutical manufacturing, and substance abuse treatment and education, serves as the Division's advisory group on matters related to prescription drug misuse. Committee members develop programs and materials to heighten the public's and health professionals' awareness of the potential dangers of prescription drugs, help assess the problems of prescription drug misuse and pill dependency in the state, and recommend strategies to help the Division address these problems.

Information on how to establish an interdisciplinary state-wide committee is available on request. Other useful resources include brochures on "Sleeping Pills and Other Choices," "Questions of Prescription Drug Misuse and Pill Dependency," "Signs of Pill Dependency," "A Guide to Wise Medication Use," and "Chemical Dependency and Women." Also available is a physician's "Desk Reference on Drug Misuse and Abuse," which contains information on "Diagnosis and Emergency Treatment," "Prescribing and Dispensing of Controlled Substances," "Special Problems of the Elderly," "General Interactions," "Street Terminology," and "Urinalysis Laboratories."

(80)

Audience	Health professions
Further Information	Controlled Substances Board 1 West Wilson Street P.O. Box 7851 Madison, Wisconsin 53707 (608) 628-5000

Resource: Conference proceedings

Drug diversion in the health professions: Progress, issues, directions. Madison, Wisconsin: Controlled Substances Board, 1983.
Drug diversion in hospitals. Madison, Wisconsin: Controlled Substances Board, 1984.

Single copies of the proceedings of Wisconsin's third and fourth conferences on diversion are available.

(81)

Audience	Professional association directors Licensing board directors Professional school deans
Further Information	Voluntary Compliance Coordinator Drug Enforcement Administration

1405 I Street, N.W.
Washington, D.C. 20537
(202) 633-1091

Resource: Conference proceedings

Konner, D. D. *Summary report: Conferences of concerned professionals allied for drug abuse prevention and control.* Unpublished conference proceedings. Washington, D.C.: Drug Enforcement Administration, 1980.

This report is the summary of proceedings of ten state voluntary compliance conferences sponsored by the DEA between 1973 and 1976. The professions involved were dentistry, medicine, nursing, pharmacy, podiatric medicine, osteopathic medicine, and veterinary medicine. Decision-makers and opinion leaders were selected from professional organizations, boards of professional licensing, and the professional schools. The report presents recommendations made by representatives of the professions on how to develop interprofessional cooperation on such problems as drug misuse, abuse, and drug diversion.

(82)

Audience	Physicians
	Pharmacists
	Law enforcement
Further Information	Coordinator
	Task Force on Prescription Drug Abuse
	California Medical Association
	44 Gough Street
	San Francisco, California 94103
	(415) 863-5522

Resource: State-wide task force/videocassettes/course

Under the auspices of the California Medical Association (CMA), a state-wide task force of physicians, pharmacists, and law enforcement representatives meets regularly to discuss common concerns about prescription drug abuse. The CMA also offers physicians a 1-day course on prescribing at its annual meeting. The course addresses issues on the interface between prescribing controls and regulatory and enforcement concerns. The CMA also has produced videocassettes on prescribing (see nos. 52, 56, and 66, above).

(83)

Audience Physicians

Further Information California Society for Treatment of Alcoholism and Other Drug Dependencies
Suite 1412
703 Market Street
San Francisco, California 94103
(415) 541-9286

Resource: Program for physicians under sanction

Since 1979, the California Society has offered a course on prescribing for physicians whose license to practice is under some sanction. A curriculum is available.

(84)

Audience Physicians

Further Information William B. Wood, MD
School of Medicine
University of North Carolina at Chapel Hill
Chapel Hill, North Carolina

Resource: Course

The School of Medicine is developing a "Special Educational Program for Physicians Requiring Review or Re-education for Professional Practice." The program will use an approach to continuing professional development that is based on constructive self-evaluation and active participation by the physician in the structuring of his or her reeducation program.

(85)

Audience Physicians

Further Information Medical Association of the State of Alabama
P.O. Box 1900-C
Montgomery, Alabama 36197
(205) 263-6441

Resource: Conference

The Alabama Governor's Conference on Drug Awareness sponsors an annual workshop on drug abuse and prescribing.

(86)
Audience Physicians

Further Information Florida Medical Association
Committee on Substance Abuse
P.O. Box 2411
Jacksonville, Florida 32203
(904) 356-1571

Resource: Conference proceedings

A conference on prescribing was held in October 1984. The State of Florida sponsored the conference in cooperation with the Florida Medical Association, other state professional associations, the American Medical Association, and the National Institute on Drug Abuse. Proceedings are available.

(87)
Audience Prescribers

Further Information South Carolina Commission on
Alcohol and Drug Abuse
Columbia, South Carolina
(803) 758-2521

Resource: Conference proceedings

The Commission's Prescription Drug Abuse Task Force hosted a March 1984 conference of southeastern state medical, pharmacy, nurses', and other health professions' societies and regulatory boards. The AMA, the National Institute on Drug Abuse, and the Drug Enforcement Administration cosponsored the conference. Proceedings are available.

(88)
Audience Physicians
Pharmacists
Dentists
Veterinarians

Further Information Director of Special Projects
Missouri Division of Alcohol
 and Drug Abuse
Department of Mental Health

2002 Missouri Boulevard
P.O. Box 687
Jefferson City, Missouri 65102
(314) 751-4122

Resource: Education program

To educate deceived practitioners, the State of Missouri and the State professional associations and boards (medicine, osteopathy, pharmacy, dentistry, veterinary medicine, nursing, and podiatry) developed a program on the problems of prescription drug abuse and the deceptive practices employed by professional patients. The "Professional Awareness Program" trains three-member teams to make presentations at regularly scheduled meetings of professional societies or hospital staff. The teams are composed of a professional practitioner, an investigator from the Missouri Bureau of Narcotics, and a member of the Missouri Task Force on Misuse, Abuse and Diversion of Prescription Drugs. Travel and other expenses are partially offset by donations from pharmaceutical firms and member associations and boards. Program materials include an "Overview Syllabus" (which describes the "Problem," Techniques of Deception," and the "Missouri Response"), "Practitioners Self-Test" of issues related to the behavior of office employees, and a "Warning" poster that outlines Missouri statutes on the use of deception or fraud.

(89)
Audience   Physicians
                      Medical educators

Further Information (See below.)

Resource: Article

Schaffner, W., Ray, W. A., Federspiel, C. F., and Miller, W. O. Improving antibiotic prescribing in office practice. *Journal of the American Medical Association*, October 7, 1983, 250 (13), 1728–1732.

"We conducted a State-wide (Tennessee) controlled trial of three methods to improve antibiotic prescribing in office practice: a mailed brochure, a drug educator visit, and a physician visit. Educational topics were three antibiotics contraindicated for office practice and oral cephalosporins. Medicaid prescribing data were used to select doctors who needed education. The effect of the methods was evaluated by comparing the change in prescribing (the year before the intervention versus the year after the intervention) for the doctors receiving education with the prescribing of comparable doctors chosen as controls. The mailed brochure had no detectable effect, and the drug educator had only a modest effect. The physician visits produced strong attributable reductions in prescribing of both drug classes. For the contraindicated antibiotics, the reductions were 18 percent in number of doctors prescribing, 44 percent in number of patients per doctor receiving these drugs, and 54 percent in number of prescriptions written per doctor. For the oral cephalosporins, both number of patients and number of prescriptions per doctor were reduced by 21 percent. Doctors responded equally well to recommendations designed to improve the quality of care and to reduce the cost of care." (Authors' Abstract)

(90)
Audience   Physicians
                         Osteopaths
                         Dentists
                         Other licensed health professionals

Further Information   Program Director
                         Mini Residency in Prescribing Controlled
                             Dangerous Substances
                         School of Osteopathic Medicine
                         Medical Arts Building
                         300 Broadway
                         Camden, New Jersey 08103
                         (609) 757-7854

Resource: Course for physicians under sanction

A "Mini Residency in Prescribing Controlled Dangerous Substances" is offered to the physician, osteopath, dentist, or other licensed health professional who wishes general information in prescribing or who has had some sanction placed against his/her license to practice. The course is scheduled for May and November 1984 in Cherry Hill and New Brunswick, New Jersey. It consists of three full days of didactic content each week for four consecutive weeks (12 days), followed by a 42-hour week clinical rotation. Topics include Pharmacology, Drugs and Drug Abuse, Pain Control, Proper Prescribing, Bioethics and Medical Ethics, Epidemiology, Behavioral Sciences, Symptomatology, Alcoholism, the Impaired Physician, and Laws and Regulations. Continuing Medical Education credits are available from the American Association of Family Physicians (62 hours), Academy of General Dentistry (72 hours), American Medical Association (Category I, 72 hours), American Osteopathic Association (Category I, 72 hours), and Academy of Medicine of New Jersey (Category I, 57 hours).

(91)
Audience   Administrators of state health departments
                         Directors of medical and pharmacy societies

Further Information   Health and Human Behavior Program
                         American Medical Association
                         535 North Dearborn Street
                         Chicago, Illinois 60610
                         (312) 645-5067

Resource: Planning guide

State program planner's resource guide. Chicago, Illinois: American Medical Association, 1985.

The guide outlines strategies and describes resources available for planning state-wide or local programs to reduce the misuse, abuse, and diversion of prescription drugs.

Index

Abortion, 48,63
Abscess, substance abuse-related,
    33,34,35,40
  of central nervous system, 51
  pulmonary, 44
Accidents, substance abuse-related,
    33,34,35,37,56
  automobile, 17
Acetaldehyde, 43,161
Acidosis, renal tubular, 104
Acupuncture, 176
Administration, of controlled substances,
    268-292
Adolescents
  alcohol abuse, 137-138,142
  drug abuse, 137-138
Adrenocortical hormone, 55
Al-Anon, 141,171
Alateen, 141,171
Alcohol
  fetal effects, 60
  as gastrointestinal cancer risk factor, 57
  hematopoietic system effects, 54
  hormonal effects, 55
  sexual functioning effects, 30-31
Alcohol abuse, see also Alcoholism
  by adolescents, 137-138,142
  breath analysis, 66-67
Alcohol history, 18-20
Alcohol intoxification, signs and symptoms,
    224-229
Alcoholics
  characteristics, 15-16
  drug abuse tendency, 20
  hospitalization, 141,151
  identification, 151
  personality types, 15
  sedative-hypnotic use, 141

Alcoholics Anonymous (A.A.),
    140-141,170-171
Alcoholism
  demographic factors, 140
  dependency testing, 65-67
  detoxification, 121
  diagnostic testing, 66-67
  liver cirrhosis and, 47
  methadone maintenance-related, 157
  overdose, 118
    signs and symptoms, 224-229
  signs and symptoms, 33-37
    direct sequelae, 33,34,35
    indirect sequelae, 34,36-37
  treatment, 140-142
    disulfiram, 161-162
    sociotherapy groups, 170-171
    tranquilizers, 162-163
  withdrawal, 119-121,123
    seizures during, 51
    signs and symptoms, 224-229
Aldehyde dehydrogenase, 161
Alkalosis, respiratory, 104
l-Alpha-Acetylmethadol, 105,116,158-159
American Medical Association, 233,236
Amphetamines
  abuse, 17,19
  behavioral effects, 53
  cardiovascular effects, 43,44
  gastrointestinal effects, 57
  neurological effects, 51
  pulmonary effects, 44
  renal effects, 56
  tolerance, 19
Analgesics
  abuse, 17,19
  for drug-dependent patients, 149,150-151
  preanesthetic, 148,149

293

renal effects, 56
withdrawal, 19
Anemia
  aplastic, 54
  megaloblastic, 54
  microangiopathic hemolytic, 55
Angel dust, *see* Phencyclidine
Angiitis, necrotizing, 56
Anoretics, *see* Appetite suppressants
Antabuse, *see* Disulfiram
Anticholinergic drugs, 43
Anticonvulsants, 57
Antipsychotic drug therapy, 95-96
Anxiety, 22,23
Anxiolytics, 17,19
Aphasia, 28
Apormorphine, 110
Appetite suppressants, 17
Arrhythmia, 43,44
  in comatose patients, 106
Arthritides, septic, 56
Assessment Interviewing Guide, 20,191-209
  patients' rationality, 200-203
  patients' readiness, 191-194
  patients' relationships, 195-200
  patients' resources, 203-209
Association of Medical Education and Research in Substance Abuse, 234,235
Ataxia, depressant-related, 53
Atrophy, cerebellar, 53
Autoimmune deficiency syndrome, 55
Automobile accidents, 17

Bacteremia, hematopoietic, 54
Bacterial infection
  cardiovascular, 42-43
  cutaneous, 34,36,40
  neurological, 51
  pulmonary, 44
"Bad trips," 129-130,169
Barbiturates
  abuse, 17
  overdose, 122
  withdrawal, 122-124
Beck Depression Inventory, 22
Beer drinker's heart, 43
Behavior modification, 176
Behavioral Assessment Inventory, 210-212
Behavioral emergencies, 94-96
Benzodiazepines
  for alcohol withdrawal, 120

  dependence, 142
  for psychiatric emergencies, 96
  withdrawal, 124,142
Beriberi heart disease, 43
Biofeedback, 176
Black Muslims, drug rehabilitation programs of, 169
Blindness, overdose-related, 50
Blocking, 27
Blood alcohol level, 12,66
Blood circulation, impairment, 56
Blood gas physiology, 104
Blood pressure
  of comatose patient, 105-106
  substance abuse-related changes, 43
Blood studies, 12,66
Brain
  degeneration, 53
  overdose sequelae, 49-50
Brain damage, thought disorders in, 27,28
Brain analysis, 66-67

Camptodactyly, 34,35,40
Candida infection, 42
Cannabis, *see* Marijuana
Cardiomyopathy, alcoholic, 43
Cardiorespiratory arrest, overdose-related, 50
Cardiovascular system
  in comatose patients, 105-106
  substance abuse effects, 42-44
Career Teacher Grants, in drug/alcohol training, 233,256-263
Catecholamines, 43,128
Cellulitis, 40
Central nervous system, abscesses, 51
Cerebellar degeneration, 53
Cerebral sequelae, of overdose, 49-50
Cerebrovascular accidents, overdose-related, 50
Certification, in drug/alcohol treatment, 235,254-256
Cheilitis, 34,36
Chlordiazepoxide
  abuse, 17
  for alcohol withdrawal, 120
Chlorpromazine, 96
Cholecystitis, 57
Chromosomal aberrations, 55
Cigarette burns, 34,36
Cigarette smoking, 18, *see also* Smoking
Circumstantiality, 27-28

Cirrhosis, hepatic, 46,47
Clinical manuals, 245-249
Clinics
 free, 169,170
 methadone, 155, *see also* Methadone maintenance
Clonidine, 176-177
Clostridium tetani, 41
Cocaine
 cardiovascular effects, 43,44
 gastrointestinal effects, 57
 neurological effects, 51
 snorting, 35
 withdrawal, 53
Codeine, abuse, 17
Coercive treatment, 171-172
Coffee drinking, 18
"Coke blues," 53
Coma
 alcohol-related, 118
 arousal measures, 103
 definition, 103
 hypoglycemic, 104
 overdose-related, 49
 phencyclidine-related, 132,133
 "shallow," 115
Comatose patient, 103-113
 cardiovascular evaluation/treatment, 105-106
 emergency treatment, 103-109,213
 evaluation, 107
 respiratory support, 103-104
Conditioned response, 25-27
Confidentiality, 12-13,141
Confrontation, 140
Constipation, 57,156
Consultations, in physician's office, 137-142
Controlled Substances Act, 235
Counseling
 in-depth, 93
 during office consultations, 137-142
Cramping, during withdrawal, 57
Criminality, heroin addiction and, 171-172
Crisis management, 93-101, *see also* Emergency treatment
 goal, 93
 guidelines, 93-94
Cross-tolerance, 123
Crush injury, 56
Curricula, for drug/alcohol training, 238-267
 development, 232-235

Cutaneous signs, of substance abuse, 33-37,39-40
 direct sequelae, 33,34,35
 indirect sequelae, 34,36-37
 septic, 39-40
Cyanide poisoning, 131
Cyclazocine, 160

Darvon, *see* Propoxylene
Darvon-N, *see* Propoxylene napsylate
Deafness, overdose-related, 50
Debilitation, substance abuse-related, 33
 pulmonary complications, 45
Delerium, post-overdose, 49-50
Delerium tremens, 119-120,121
Delusions, 27
Demerol, *see* Meperidine
Denial, 140
Dental disorders, 34,36
Dentists
 impaired, 284-285
 training resources, 284-285, 289-290, 291-292
Dependence
 definition, 12-13
 psychological vs. physical, 63
 tolerance and, 64
Depressants
 dependency testing, 64
 intoxification, signs and symptoms, 224-229
 neurological effects, 53
 overdose, 121-122
  pulmonary effects, 44-45
  signs and symptoms, 224-229
 sexual functioning effects, 30,47
 withdrawal, 122-123
  signs and symptoms, 224-229
Dermatitis, 34,35,36,40
Dermatological complications
 dermatitis, 34,35,36,40
 physical examination for, 33-37
 pruritus, 34,40
 septic cutaneous, 39-40
Detoxification
 alcohol, 121
 definition, 12
 FDA regulations, 156
 heroin/methadone, 117
Diabetes, 55,57
Diagnosis, of substance abuse
 in emergency treatment, 98-99

of medical complications, 11-12,39-61
patient interview in, 15-31
    orientation to patient, 15-18
    personal history, 18-31
physical examination in, 33-37
posttest, 69-78
pretest, 1-10
terminology, 12-13
Diagnostic aids, 214-223
    for hallucinogen intoxification, 217
    for opiate abuse
        intoxification/overdose, 222
        withdrawal, 223
    for phencyclidine intoxification/overdose, 218-219
    for sedatives-hypnotics abuse
        intoxification/overdose, 220
        withdrawal, 221
    for stimulants abuse
        intoxification/overdose, 215
        withdrawal, 216
Diagnostic tests, 63-68
    alcohol dependency, 65-67
    evaluation, 67-68
    laboratory, 66-67
    nalorphine, 63
    naloxone, 63-65
    recommended, 12
Diarrhea, 57
Diazepam
    abuse, 17
    for alcoholism treatment, 162
    dependence, 19
    half-life, 100-101
    for hyperventilation management, 100-101
    impulse control and, 96
    for seizure management, 108
    withdrawal, 142
        seizures during, 51
Diederich, Charles, 165
Dihydromorphinone, 146,150,151
Dilantin, see Phenytoin
Dilaudid, see Dihydromorphinone
Dispensing, training resources for, 268-292
Disulfiram, 161-162
Dolophine, see Methadone
Doriden, see Glutethimide
Drop-in centers, 169-170
Drug abuse
    by adolescents, 137-138
    maternal, 48-49,58-60

patient's unawareness of, 19
signs and symptoms, 33-37
    direct sequelae, 33,34,35
    indirect sequelae, 34,36-37
Drug addicts
    alcohol abuse tendency, 20
    attitudes towards physicians, 138-139
    characteristics, 15-16
    personality types, 15
    pregnancy of, 48-49,58-60
    psychological characteristics, 15
    sexual functioning, 30-31
    surgery, 148-150
Drug adulterants, see also Quinine; Talc
    pulmonary effects, 44
Drug Enforcement Administration, 235-236
Drug history, 18-20

Edema
    cutaneous, 33,34,35
    pulmonary, 45,149
Educational resources, see Training resources
Electrocardiogram, 12,66
    of comatose patients, 106
Electroencephalogram, 12,53
Emergency treatment, 93-101
    behavioral, 94-96
    comatose patients, 103-109,213
        cardiovascular evaluation/treatment, 105-106
        evaluation, 107
        naloxone administration, 105
        respiratory support, 103-104
    diagnostic procedures, 98-99
    fever of unknown origin, 214
    guidelines, 93-94
    hyperventilation, 100-101
    observation procedures, 98-99
    overdose, 213
    in physician's office, 138
    seizures, 107-109
    semicomatose patient, 109-113
        emesis, 109,110
        gastric lavage, 111-113
    shock, 99-100
    suicidal patients, 97
    violent patients, 96-97
Emesis, see Vomiting
Encephalopathy, 53
Encounter groups, 166
Endocarditis, 42-43,51

Endocrine function, 55
Epilepsy, 57
  seizures, 107,108
Epinephrine, 55
Examinations, for drug/alcohol treatment certification, 254-256

Family, involvement in treatment, 141
Fatty liver, 47
Fetal alcohol syndrome, 60
Fetus
  maternal alcohol use effects, 60
  maternal marijuana use effects, 60
  methadone dependency, 48-49,156-157
  withdrawal, 58
Fever of unknown origin, 214
Films, for drug/alcohol training, 249-254
Fixed drug eruption, 34,35
Flashbacks, 130
Flight of ideas, 28
Food and Drug Administration, 150,156
Fractures, 56
Frostbite, 56

Gamma glutamyltranspeptidase test, 47,65-66
Gangrene, 34,35,56
Ganja, 134
Gasoline sniffing, 53
Gastric lavage, 111-113
  of comatose patient, 106
Gastrointestinal system complications, 57
GGT test, see Gamma glutamyltranspeptidase test
Glomerulonephritis, 56
Glucose, intravenous administration, 104,105
Glue sniffing, 36,43
Glutethimide
  abuse, 17
  overdose, 109,122
  withdrawal, 123
Gonorrhea, 47,66
Gordon test, 22
Gram-negative bacterial infection, 42
Grand mal seizure, 107,120
Growth hormone, 55

Haldol, see Haloperidol
Hallucinations
  alcoholic auditory, 119
  cardiovascular effects, 43
  definition, 27

Hallucinogens
  clinical signs, 129-130
  diagnostic aids, 217
  flashbacks, 130
  gastrointestinal effects, 57
  intoxification, signs and symptoms, 217,224-229
  overdose
    neurological complications, 51
    signs and symptoms, 224-229
  renal effects, 56
  withdrawal, 224-229
Haloperidol, 96,121
Hash oil, 134
Hashish, 134
Health professionals, training resources, 231-292
Heart failure, congestive, 149
Hematopoietic system complications, 54-55
Hemiballistic movements, 50
Hepatitis, 45-47
  Australia antigen detection, 46,47
  neurological complications, 51
Heroin, see also Methadone; Methadone maintenance
  adulterants, 41,50,145,146
  excretion, 145-146
  snorting, 35,45-46
Heroin abuse
  cardiovascular complications, 42-43
  criminality and, 171-172
  coercive treatment, 171-172
  dependency testing, 64-65
  detoxification, 117
  hepatitis and, 45-46
  neonatal withdrawal, 59-60
  nephrotic syndrome, 49,56
  overdose
    neurological complications, 49-50
    pulmonary complications, 44-45
  pentazocine abuse and, 125
  polydrug dependency and, 116-117
  during pregnancy, 58-59
  prematurity and, 59
  tetanus and, 41
  withdrawal, 154
Himmelsbach Rating Scale, 63
Hormones, drug interactions, 55
Hospitalization
  of alcoholics, 141,151
  of opiate-dependent patients, 143-152
    analgesia for, 149,150-151

methadone maintenance for, 143-145
neonatal withdrawal syndrome
   management, 151
"street addicts," 145-148
surgery for, 148-150
Hotlines, 169,170
Hypertension, 43,44
   in comatose patients, 105-106
   phencyclidine-related, 133
   pulmonary, 44
   stimulant effects, 58
Hyperventilation, management, 100-101
Hypnotics, see Sedative-hypnotics
Hypoglycemia, alcoholic, 55
Hypotension
   in comatose patients, 106
   preanesthetic, 148
Hypoxia, overdose-related, 107-108

Ileus, postoperative, 149
Immune system
   alcohol effects, 54
   drug effects, 54-55
Immunoassay, 67
Immunoglobulins
   in nephrotic syndrome, 56
   intravenous drug infection effects, 54-55
Impulse control, 24,96
Incoherence, 28
Indicators, of substance abuse, 16-17
Infection, see also Bacterial infection
   intraarterial, 56
   neurological, 51
Inhalation, of drugs, 54
Insulin, 55,57
Intellectualization, 27
Intoxification, signs and symptoms, 224-229
Intraarterial infection, 56
Intraarterial injection, 40
Intravenous injection
   bacteremia from, 54
   immunoglobulin response, 54-55
   pulmonary complications, 44-45
   skin tracks from, 33,34,35
   tourniquet pigmentation from, 34,36
Intubation, endotracheal, 104
Ipecac, 110

Jaundice, 34,36
Judgement disturbances, 28-29

Laboratory tests, 66-67
Law enforcement personnel, training
   resources, 274-275,287-288
Librarians
   Substance Abuse Librarians Information
      Service, 234-235
   training resources, 243-244
Librium, see Chlordiazepoxide
Lithium
   abuse, 21
   for alcoholism treatment, 162,163
Liver cancer, 47
Liver disease, 45-47
   cirrhosis, 46,47
   encephalopathy, 53
   in surgical patients, 149
Lorazepam, 120
Low back pain, 56
Low birth weight, 59,60
LSD, see Lysergic acid diethylamide
Lymphadenopathy, 54
Lysergic acid diethylamide (LSD)
   chromosomal effects, 55
   overdose, 51

Macrocytosis, in alcoholism, 66
Malabsorption, in alcoholism, 57
Malaria, 41
Malnutrition
   alcoholism-related, 53,57,108
   drug abuse-related, 57,108
   vitamin therapy, 108
Manic-depressive illness, 21
Marchiafava-Bignami disease, 53
Marijuana, see also Tetrahydrocannabinol
   adverse effects, 134-135
   cardiovascular effects, 43
   fetal effects, 60
   hematopoietic system effects, 55
   reproductive system effects, 30
   sexual functioning effects, 47-48
Medical complications, of substance abuse,
   39-61
   cardiovascular, 42-44
   dermatological, 39-40
   diagnosis, 11-12
   endocrine, 55
   gastrointestinal, 57
   hematopoietic, 54-55
   hepatic, 45-47
   malaria, 41

neuromuscular, 49-53
physical examination, 33-37
preexisting conditions, 57-58
during pregnancy, 58-59
pulmonary, 44-45
renal, 56
reproductive, 47-49
skeletal, 56
tetanus, 41
Medical educators, training resources, 238,240-242,244-245,254-255,256-266,279-280,286-287,290-292
Medical history, 98
Medical Monograph Series, The, 233-234
Meningitis
bacterial, 51
pneumococcal, 43
Menstruation, drug abuse effects, 48
Mental status examination, 95,96
Meperidine, 150,151
Methadone
characteristics, 153-154
definition, 13
dependency testing, 64-65
detoxification, 117
dosage, 154-155
fetal effects, 48-49,156-157
gastrointestinal effects, 57
neonatal dependence, 59
overdose
observation period, 105
pulmonary effects, 45
sexual functioning effects, 30
side effects, 156
withdrawal, 117,153-154
Methadone maintenance, 153-158
efficacy, 154,158
eligibility for, 156
FDA regulations, 150,156
on general medical wards, 143-145
during pregnancy, 48-49,59,156-157
problems, 156-158
programs, 155
psychotherapy and, 155-156
for "street addicts," 145-147
for surgical patients, 148-149,150
urinalysis monitoring, 155
Methaqualone
abuse, 17
overdose, 122
withdrawal, 122-123

Methylphenidate
pentazocine abuse and, 125
pulmonary effects, 44
Michigan Alcoholism Screening Test (MAST), 65,140
Minnesota Multiphasic Personality Inventory (MMPI), 21-22
Minors, *see also* Adolescents
treatment, 138
Minor-tranquilizers, *see* Depressants
Miosis, 115
Mononeuropathy, atraumatic, 50
Mood disturbance assessment, 22-23
Morphine
as analgesic, 150-151
dependency testing, 64-65
excretion, 145-146
Myelitis, transverse, 49,50
Myocardial disease, 43
Myopathy
alcoholic, 49
chronic fibrosing, 50-51
unilateral, 51

Nalorphine test, 63
Naloxone
for comatose patients, 105
for opiate abuse, 115,116,160
for physician's office emergencies, 138
Naloxone test, 63-65
Naltrexone, 160-161
Narcotic-antagonists, 160-161
for opiate overdose, 115-116
National Clearinghouse for Alcohol Information, 139
National Clearinghouse for Drug Abuse Information, 139
National Council on Alcoholism, 232
National Institute on Alcohol Abuse and Alcoholism, 233,234,235
National Institute on Drug Abuse, 233,235
Nausea, drug-related, 57
Necrosis, hepatic, 47
Needle-track scars, 33,34,35,39-40
Neonatal withdrawal syndrome, 59-60,151
Neonate, methadone-dependent, 59
Nephrotic syndrome, 49,56
Nerve lesions, peripheral, 50
Neuromuscular complications, 49-53
infectious, 51
noninfectious, 49-51

of non-opiate drugs, 51-53
postinfectious, 51
NIMH 35-Item Symptom Rating Scale, 22
Nurses
 impaired, 283-284
 training resources, 239-240,246,251,
  268-269,283-284
Nystagmus, 53

Obsession, 28
Opiates
 dependency testing, 63-65,67
 endocrine function effects, 55
 gastrointestinal effects, 57
 intoxification
  diagnostic aids, 222
  signs and symptoms, 222,224-229
 overdose
  coma, 115
  diagnostic aids, 222
  signs and symptoms, 222,224-229
  treatment, 115-116
 pulmonary effects, 45
 sexual functioning effects, 30
 withdrawal, 116-117
  clonidine for, 176-177
  diagnostic aids, 223
  signs and symptoms, 146,223,224-229
Organizations, for drug/alcohol training,
  256-267
Orientation
 disturbances, 26,28
 testing, 95
Osteomyelitis, 56
Overdose
 alcohol, 118,224-229
 depressants, 44-45,121-122,224-229
 emergency treatment, 138,213
 hypoxia during, 107-108
 neurological complications, 49-50,51,53
 opiates, 115-116,222,224-229
 phencyclidine, 218-219
 physician's office emergency treatment,
  138
 pulmonary effects, 44-45
 renal failure from, 56
 sedative-hypnotics, 121-122,220
 seizures during, 51,107-108
 signs and symptoms, 224-229
 stimulants, 128,215
 tricyclic antidepressants, 124-125
Oxazepam, 120

Pain, abdominal, 58
Pancreatitis, 57
Panic, 130,134
Pap smear, 12,66
Parents, of drug-abusing adolescents,
  137-138
Parkinson's syndrome, 50
Passivity, 15
Patient interview, 15-31, *see also*
   Assessment Interviewing Guide
 components, 11
 false information in, 29
 orientation to patient, 15-18
 personal history, 18-31
  checklist, 26,29
  drug/alcohol history, 18-20
  psychiatric problems, 22-29
  psychological functioning assessment,
   21-29
  psychological tests, 21-22
  sexual functioning assessment, 30-31
  social functioning assessment, 20
Patient records, confidentiality of, 13-14,
  141
PCP, *see* Phencyclidine
Pellagra, 53
Pentazocine
 abuse, 17,125-126
 contraindications, 149,151
Pentobarbital, for barbiturate withdrawal,
  123
Peptic ulcer, 57
Perseveration, 28
Personal history interview, 18-31
 drug/alcohol history, 18-20
 false information in, 29
 psychological functioning assessment,
  21-29
  checklist, 26,29
  psychiatric problems, 22-29
  psychological tests, 21-22
  sexual functioning assessment, 30-31
  social functioning assessment, 20
Personality types, of substance abusers, 15
Pharmacists
 impaired, 282-283
 training resources, 268-269,272-273,278,
  279,282-283,284-285,287,289-290
Pharmacotherapy, 153-163
 l-alpha-acetylmethadol, 105,116,158-159
 disulfiram, 161-162
 methadone maintenance, 153-158

narcotic antagonists, 160-161
propoxyphene napsylate, 159-160
Phencyclidine
  adulterants, 131
  hypertensive effects, 44
  intoxification
    diagnostic aids, 67,218-219
    signs and symptoms, 218-219,224-229
  neurological effects, 53
  overdose
    diagnostic aids, 218-219
    neurological complications, 51
    signs and symptoms, 218-219,224-229
  reactions, 131-134
  withdrawal, 224-229
Phenobarbital, 123-124
Phenytoin, 108
Physical examination, 33-37
  components, 11
  in emergency treatment, 98-99
Physician(s)
  drug addicts' attitudes towards, 138-139
  impaired, 140
  orientation to patient, 15-18
  patient confidentiality and, 13-14,141
  training resources, 231-292
Physician assistants, training resources, 248-249,269-270
Physician's office, drug/alcohol treatment in, 137-142
Piloerection, 37
Placental transport, of drugs, 48, *see also* Pregnancy
Pleasure seeking, 16
Plexitis, 49
Pneumonia, 42,43
  aspiration, 45
Polyarteritis, 43
Polydrug abuse
  by heroin addicts, 116-117
  psychological disturbances and, 21
  treatment, 135,142
    sociotherapy, 169
  withdrawal, 135
Polyneuropathy, 53
Pregnancy
  in drug abusers, 48-49,58-59
  methadone maintenance during, 48-49,59,156-157
  naloxone testing avoidance during, 63
  testing, 12,66
Prematurity, 59,157

Prescribing, training resources, 235-236,268-292
Prescription drugs
  abuse, 17
  patients' use of, 18
Prisons, coercive drug treatment in, 172
Propoxyphene
  abuse, 17
  treatment, 126
  overdose, pulmonary effects, 45
Propoxyphene napsylate, 159-160
Pruritis, 34,40
Psychiatric examination, 95,96
Psychiatric problems, 22-29
  emergency treatment, 94-96
  hallucinogen-related, 129-130
Psychiatrists, training resources, 239
Psychoanalysis, 93
Psychological functioning assessment, 21-29
Psychological illness, treatment outcome and, 21
Psychological tests, 21-22
Psychologists, training resources, 246
Psychotherapeutic drugs, 21
Psychotherapy, 21,93
  for methadone maintenance patients, 155-156
Pulmonary complications, 44-45
Puncture marks, 33,34,35,39-40
Pupillary conditions, in overdose, 99,115
Pyribenzamine, *see* Tripelennamine

Quaalude, *see* Methaqualone
Quinine, as heroin adulterant, 41,50
  urinary excretion, 145,146

Rationality assessment, 17,200-203
Rehabilitation, *see also* Sociotherapy
  definition, 13
Relaxation techniques, 176
Renal complications, 56
Renal failure, 56
Reproductive system complications, 47-49
Respiratory support, for comatose patients, 103-104
Reviews, of drug/alcohol training resources, 238-267
Rhabdomyolysis, acute, 49,50
Ritalin, *see* Methylphenidate
"Rum fits," 120

Salicylates, 54
Secobarbital, 123
Schizophrenia, 27,28
Sedative-hypnotics
  abuse, 17
  alcohol abuse and, 141
  dependence-producing dosages, 52,53
  intoxification
    diagnostic tests, 67,220
    signs and symptoms, 220
  overdose, 121-122
    diagnostic aids, 220
    signs and symptoms, 220
    for psychiatric emergencies, 95-96
  withdrawal, 122-123
    diagnostic aids, 221
    signs and symptoms, 221
Seizures
  alcohol-related, 120
  convulsive, 49
  differentiation, 51,53
  epileptic, 107,108
  grand mal, 107,120
  management, 107-109
  overdose-related, 51,107-108
  as substance abuse indicator, 17
  during withdrawal, 51,53,107,108
Semicomatose patients, 109-113
  emesis, 109,110
  gastric lavage, 111-113
Sensorium orientation, 26,28
Serological tests, 12,66-67
Serratia marcescens, 54
Serum glutamic-pyruvic transaminase test (SGOT), 66
Sexual functioning, 47-48,55, *see also* Reproductive system complications
  assessment, 30-31
SGOT test, *see* Serum glutamic-pyruvic transaminase test
Shock
  in comatose patient, 106
  management, 99-100
  in sedative-hypnotic overdose, 122
Signs, of substance abuse, 33-37
  definition, 13
  direct sequelae, 33,34,35
  hallucinogen intoxification, 217
  indirect sequelae, 34,36-37
  intoxification, 224-229
  opiate abuse

    intoxification/overdose, 222
    withdrawal, 223
  overdose, 224-229
  phencyclidine abuse, 218-219
  sedative-hypnotic abuse
    intoxification/overdose, 220
    withdrawal, 221
  stimulant abuse
    intoxification/overdose, 215
    withdrawal, 126
  withdrawal, 224-229
Skeletal system complications, 56
Skin popping, 34,35,41
Skin tracks, 33,34,35,39-40
Sleeping pills, 19
SMA-6 serological test, 12,67
SMA-12 serological test, 12,66,67
Smoking, 18,45,57
Social functioning assessment, 20
Sociotherapy, 17,165-173
  for alcoholism, 170-171
  coercive treatment, 171-172
  drop-in centers, 169-170
  free clinics, 169,170
  hotlines, 169,170
  religious-oriented, 169
  therapeutic communities, 165-169
    modified, 168-169
Solvents
  hematopoietic system effects, 54
  neurological effects, 53
Staphylococcal infections
  cardiovascular, 42,43
  cutaneous, 36
  respiratory, 43
State-wide programs, in drug/alcohol training, 285-292
Status epilepticus, 49,108,133
Status inversion, 138-139
Steatorrhea, 57
Steatosis, hepatic, 47
Stimulants
  abuse, 17
    symptoms, 127-128
  chronic abuse syndrome, 128
  gastrointestinal effects, 57
  hypertensive effects, 58
  intoxification
    diagnostic tests, 67
    signs and symptoms, 224-229
  overdose, 128

diagnostic aids, 215
  signs and symptoms, 215,224-229
  sexual functioning effects, 30,47-48
  withdrawal, 128-129
    diagnostic aids, 216
    signs and symptoms, 216,224-229
Stream-of-thought disturbances, 27-28
"Street addicts," on general medical ward, 145-148
Stress
  hormones and, 55
  treatment, 16
Subcutaneous injection
  pop scars from, 34,35
  tetanus from, 41
Substance abuse, see also Alcohol abuse; Alcoholism; Drug abuse; specific substances of abuse
  indicators, 16-17
  signs and symptoms, 33-37
Substance Abuse Librarians Information Service, 234-235
Succinylcholine chloride, 103-104
Sudden death, 43
Suicidal patients
  management, 97
  wrist scars, 36
Suicide potential assessment, 23-24
Surgery, on substance abusers, 148-150
Symptoms, of substance abuse, 33-37
  definition, 13
  direct sequelae, 33,34,35
  hallucinogen intoxification, 217
  indirect sequelae, 34,36-37
  intoxification, 224-229
  opiate abuse, 146
    intoxification/overdose, 222
    withdrawal, 223
  overdose, 224-229
  phencyclidine intoxification/overdose, 218-219
  sedative-hypnotic intoxification/overdose, 220,221
  stimulants abuse
    intoxification/overdose, 215
    withdrawal, 216
  withdrawal, 224-229
Synanon, 165

Tachyarrythmia, 43
Talc, as drug adulterant, 44,50

Talwin, see Pentazocine
Tangential thinking, 28
Tattoos, 34,35,36
Teen Challenge, 169
Testosterone, 47,55
Tetanus, 41
Tetrahydrocannabinol, 67,131
THC, see Tetrahydrocannabinol
Therapeutic communities, 165-169
  modified, 168-169
Thiamine deficiency, 43
Thorazine, see Chlorpromazine
Thought disorders, 26,27-29
  characterization, 27-29
  content disturbances, 28
  definition, 27
  medication, 96
  patient interview checklist of, 26
Tolerance, physical dependence and, 64
Tourniquet pigmentation, 34,36
Training resources, for drug/alcohol treatment, 231-292
  administration of controlled substances, 268-292
  Career Teacher Grants, 233,256-263
  certification procedures, 254-256
  clinical manuals, 245-249
  curricula, 232-235,238-267
  for dentists, 284-285,289-290,291-292
  dispensation of controlled substances, 268-292
  drug diversion for abuse, 274-280
  educational, 231-267
  examinations, 254-256
  films, 249-254
  general reviews, 238-267
  historical development, 232-236
  for impaired professionals, 280-285
  for law enforcement personnel, 274-275,287-288
  for librarians, 243-244
  for medical educators, 238,240-242, 244-245,254-255,256-266,279-280, 286-287,290-292
  for nurses, 239-240,246,251,268-269, 283-284
  organizations, 256-268
  for pharmacists, 268-269,272-273,278, 279,282-283,284-285,287,289-290
  for physician assistants, 248-249,269-270
  for physicians, 238-292

prescription of controlled substances,
    268-292
  for psychiatrists, 239
  for psychologists, 246
  state-wide programs, 285-292
  for veterinarians, 289-290
  videocassettes, 249-254
Tranquilizers, see also Depressants
  for alcoholism treatment, 162-163
Transcendental meditation, 175
Trauma
  accident-related, 33
  alcoholism-related, 56
  as substance abuse indicator, 17
  surgical, 148
Treatment, see also Emergency treatment
  alcohol overdose, 118
  alcohol withdrawal, 119-120
  depressant overdose, 121-122
  depressant withdrawal, 122-124
  experimental modalities, 175-177
  hallucinogen abuse, 129-131
  individualized approach, 16
  information sources, 139-140
  long-term, 13
  marijuana abuse, 134-135
  methadone withdrawal, 117
  opiate overdose, 115-116
  opiate withdrawal, 116-117
  patient confidentiality restrictions and,
    13-14,141
  pentazocine abuse, 125-126
  pharmacotherapy, 153-163
  phencyclidine abuse, 131-134
  polydrug abuse, 135
  posttest, 179-189
  pretest, 79-91
  propoxyphene abuse, 126
  sedative-hypnotic overdose, 121-122
  sedative-hypnotic withdrawal, 122-124
  short-term, 13
  sociotherapy, 165-173
  stimulants abuse, 127-128
  stimulants withdrawal, 128-129
  stress, 16
  terminology, 12-13
  tricyclic antidepressant overdose, 124-125
  volatiles abuse, 126-127
Treatment outcome, psychological illness
    and, 21
Tricyclic antidepressants
  for alcoholism, 163

  cardiovascular effects, 43-44
  overdose, 124-125
Triglycerides, in alcoholism, 66
Tripelennamine, 125
"T's and Blues," 125
Tuberculosis, 45

Ulceration
  cutaneous, 33,34,35
  peptic, 57
Unconsciousness, see also Coma; Comatose
    patient
  injuries acquired during, 56
Uric acid level, in alcoholism, 66
Urinalysis, 12
  as drug use indicator, 20,66,155
  for morphine, 145-146
  for opiates, 63,64
  for quinine, 145,146
  as social functioning indicator, 20

Valium, see Diazepam
Vascular changes, substance abuse-related,
    43-44
Venereal disease, 47,58
Veterinarians, training resources, 289-290
Videocassettes, for drug/alcohol training,
    249-254
Violence potential assessment, 24-25
Violent patients, mamagement, 96-97
Vitamin therapy, 108
Volatile nitrites, 47-48
Volatiles, abuse, 126-127
Vomiting
  drug abuse-related, 57
  by overdose patients, 109,110
  phencyclidine-related, 131,132

Wernicke-Korsakoff syndrome, 53
Withdrawal, see also Detoxification
  alcohol, 51,119-121,123,224-229
  analgesics, 19
  benzodiazepines, 124,142
  cocaine, 53
  depressants, 122-123,224-229
  diazepam, 51,142
  in epileptics, 57
  fetal, 58
  gastrointestinal effects, 57
  heroin, 154
  methadone, 117,153-154
  neonatal, 59-60,151

opiates, 116-117,146,176-177,223, 224-229
polydrug abuse, 135
propoxyphene, 126
sedative-hypnotics, 122-123,221
seizures during, 51,53,107,108
signs and symptoms, 224-229
stimulants, 128-129,216
substitution technique, 123-124
Wonderlic test, 22

Zung test, 22